Psychiatry of Pandemics

Damir Huremović
Editor

Psychiatry of Pandemics

A Mental Health Response
to Infection Outbreak

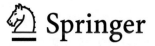 Springer

Editor
Damir Huremović
North Shore University Hospital
Manhasset, NY
USA

ISBN 978-3-030-15345-8   ISBN 978-3-030-15346-5   (eBook)
https://doi.org/10.1007/978-3-030-15346-5

This Springer imprint is published by the registered company Springer Nature Switzerland AG
The registered company address is: Gewerbestrasse 11, 6330 Cham, Switzerland

Preface

This book could have been written a century ago – at a time when the last true pandemic was sweeping the globe and psychiatry was emerging from the confines of insanity asylums and establishing itself as a reputable medical specialty. At the time, it did not happen, and for the next hundred years or so, psychiatry would not seriously consider and address the mental health challenges accompanying massive infectious disease outbreaks and pandemics.

As the public anxieties about infectious disease outbreaks rose in recent years with the advent of SARS, N1H1 flu, Ebola, and Zika, we observed in awe how the public would react to an impending outbreak in their midst and how those public fears would emerge and spread like, well, an epidemic. A wave of public angst anticipating an outbreak would swell, crest, and then subside, very much like the wave of the infection outbreak itself. In the wake of both waves, relief would follow.

While the aftermath of an outbreak would bestow on us serious consequences, but also newly acquired knowledge and immunity, the aftermath of an emotional outbreak would bequeath to us mostly oblivion. Content that a crisis was avoided or prevented, individuals and communities alike would long to return to their daily routines and banish *the plague* from their conscious thoughts.

This process of etching the memory of a disease into our antibodies, yet erasing it from our thoughts, appears to be natural and to foster self-preservation. Few human experiences are so profound and so terrifying, as is the fear of being stricken by a grave *contagion*, a process that can not only kill us, but worse – it can mutilate our body and transmogrify our soul into something no longer recognizable, no longer human. This notion is only made worse by the realization that such affliction is passed onto us by our fellow humans, even our loved ones, or that we have passed it onto them. Such realization poisons and unravels the social fabric of humanity.

It is, therefore, understandable that the dread surrounding a severe contagious outbreak cannot be tolerated for long and needs to be banished from our individual and collective *conscious*. One can appreciate how beneficial and comforting oblivion may be for the survivors of an outbreak. This appreciation, however, should not prevent us, scientists and medical professionals, from exploring this very matter, seeking a deeper understanding. And that was why we ventured to write this book, a book perhaps a hundred years overdue.

For us, compiling this manuscript was a series of journeys – a journey through the history of medicine and humankind, a journey through depths of human psyche, a journey through vast expanses of pharmacology, a brief excursion into legal frameworks and international treaties, an exploration of the role of social media and so on; in a way, this text is a collection of souvenirs we brought back from those journeys.

We dedicate this book to all the brave individuals, legendary and unknown, who devoted their lifetimes and sometimes sacrificed their lives fighting infections, studying illnesses, and advancing the health of humankind.

We dedicate it to our mentors and our teachers, who taught us medicine and psychiatry, and then pushed us forward and challenged us to aim high seeking knowledge and understanding.

We dedicate this book to our families whose love, understanding, and selfless support translated into precious time we needed for research and writing.

We hope you enjoy the journey.

Manhasset, NY, USA   Damir Huremović

Contents

Contributors

Saeed Ahmed, MD Department of Psychiatry, Nassau University Medical Center, East Meadow, NY, USA

Christy Duan, MD Department of Psychiatry, Zucker Hillside Hospital, Astoria, NY, USA

Damir Huremović, MD, MPP, FAPA, FACLP North Shore University Hospital, Manhasset, NY, USA

Saira Hussain, DO Department of Psychiatry, North Shore University Hospital, Manhasset, NY, USA

Sameer Khan, MD Department of Psychiatry, Private Practice, New York, NY, USA

Jacqueline Levin, MD Department of Psychiatry, North Shore University Hospital, Manhasset, NY, USA

Howard Linder, MD, FAPA, FACLP Department of Psychiatry, Zucker Hillside Hospital, Glen Oaks, NY, USA

Guitelle St. Victor, MD, FAPA, FACLP Department of Psychiatry, Nassau University Medical Center, East Meadow, NY, USA

Chapter 1
Introduction

Damir Huremović

Catastrophic pandemics have been occurring at regular intervals throughout human history, with the last one (Spanish flu pandemic of 1918) taking place a century ago, just before the advent of modern psychiatry as a science and a clinical specialty. As a consequence, contemporary psychiatry had little opportunity to seriously consider such historically important phenomena through its clinical, scientific lens. At least in part, an explanation for this may lie in the distribution of pathologies and resources – with an exception of HIV epidemic and seasonal flu pandemics, infectious disease outbreaks, and their burden remains limited to developing countries, tying up their national and international (where available) healthcare resources. Developed countries, on the other hand, have managed to significantly ameliorate the burden of infectious diseases and minimize possibilities of an outbreak through improvements in standard of living, general precautions, and immunization. With communicable diseases not among the

D. Huremović (✉)
North Shore University Hospital, Manhasset, NY, USA
e-mail: dhuremov@northwell.edu

© Springer Nature Switzerland AG 2019
D. Huremović (ed.), *Psychiatry of Pandemics*,
https://doi.org/10.1007/978-3-030-15346-5_1

first five causes of death in the developed world [1], it is understandable that research interest in infectious diseases and, particularly, in pandemic outbreaks, remains marginal within all specialties not directly involved in combating communicable diseases.

Some recent events, however, including outbreaks of Zika virus and MERS and, prior to that, outbreaks of Ebola hemorrhagic fever and SARS, have managed to draw global attention to a possibility of a real pandemic in the twenty-first century, stirring up anxiety and uneasiness in societies, developed and developing alike, across the globe. Despite advances in healthcare technologies, therapeutics, and international surveillance efforts, a catastrophic outbreak of pandemic proportions remains a faint, but distinct possibility [2]. Human impact on global biosphere, population growth, expansion of international travel and trade, armed conflicts, misuse of antimicrobial agents, and changes in attitudes toward immunization, all increase the odds of such an outbreak occurring spontaneously. In a more sinister scenario, sadly, a pandemic outbreak can be intentionally instigated by state or non-state actors through acts of deliberately orchestrated biological warfare and bioterrorism [3]. In order to be able to adequately respond to such global health challenges, the international public health community seeks to identify infectious diseases that can pose a public health risk because of their epidemic potential and for which there are no countermeasures or they remain woefully insufficient ("Disease X", per WHO terminology) [4]. Participation of mental health experts in projects devoted to preparing for a pandemic outbreak remains negligible or very limited [5].

Approaches to mental health and psychiatric care in such outbreaks remain poorly understood [6], outlined, or covered by existing interests, research, and literature within psychiatry as a discipline. Moreover, it is unclear what part of psychiatry could and should "claim" such infectious outbreaks as its legitimate study subject; two subspecialties within psychiatry could stake such claim, but neither fully does.

One such subspecialty of psychiatry – Consultation Liaison psychiatry (CLP) – addresses the interface between mental health and other medical specialties, including infectious diseases. Most mental health resources and research dedicated to the area of infectious diseases within CLP are, however, largely focused on infections that endemically impose steady and significant public health burden on societies (e.g., HIV, Hepatitis C, or TB). With their steady and predictable epidemiology, such diseases allow for studious and systematic approach which has been utilized over the past decades. This includes neuropsychiatric sequelae, emotional burden, social stigma, and impact on communities. Within this branch, unfortunately, there is virtually no substantial knowledge, focus, or interest in rapidly spreading outbreaks of infectious diseases that leave little time to studiously and fully comprehend mental health aspects of such illnesses, with potentially devastating social impact, both during the outbreaks and in their aftermath.

In those instances, another subspecialty of psychiatry – disaster psychiatry – lends itself as a primary discipline to outline mental health responses that are, by default, undertaken as emergency mental health responses to a disaster. While the general approach of disaster psychiatry is applicable to organizing and providing emergency mental health response to epidemic outbreaks, there is little focus within disaster psychiatry on infectious diseases alone. While this general approach to mental health in a disaster can also be used in cases of infectious diseases outbreaks, there are several crucial idiosyncrasies in pandemic mental health that make it stand out and make it worth a more serious consideration in literature and research.

Unique features of mental health responses in pandemic outbreaks include the following:

- Time lapse and disease modeling – Pandemic outbreaks, unlike most disasters, have predictable epidemiological models that allow limited, but valuable, time for prognostication, planning, and preparation as the pandemic approaches and progresses.
- Mental health burden on health workers – Health workers in pandemic outbreaks are both at increased risk for

infection and psychological trauma while caring for infected patients, with rates of PTSD among healthcare personnel in such situations reaching 20 percent, as was the case during the 2003 SARS outbreak [7].

- Quarantine - For centuries, a routinely practiced method of infection control, quarantine and, overall, social distancing have received surprisingly little attention in psychiatric literature so far. Prolonged isolation and separation from families and their community can nevertheless have profound effects on individuals even if they are merely isolated and not directly affected by the disease. Similar effects can be observed in healthcare workers placed in isolation. Quarantine and isolation warrant special mental health attention in any infectious disease outbreak.

- Neuropsychiatric sequelae among survivors – Neuropsychiatric sequelae of surviving an infectious illness, its complications, and complications associated with treatment may warrant sustained mental health focus and attention. This set of sequelae may require an expansion in resources and expertise from more trauma-focused to include neuropsychiatric aspects of care in order to prevent and minimize long-term disabilities.

- Behavioral contagion and emotional epidemiology – Managing concerns, fears, and misconceptions at the local community and broader public level become as important as treating individual patients. Mental health providers may find themselves participating in public mental health activities, helping to formulate responses to alleviate public anxiety and concerns; basic understanding of *emotional epidemiology* can be helpful in such situations [8].

- Precarious status of healthcare facilities and healthcare workers – In the midst of a pandemic outbreak and unlike in other disasters, healthcare facilities may transform from points of care to nodes of transmission, further jeopardizing public trust in the healthcare system and its ability to respond to the outbreak. Understanding, for example, the emotional burden on healthcare workers, exposed to disease and separated from families, or challenges surrounding immunization hesitancy in a particular community may help mental health providers play an instrumental role on a multidisciplinary public health team deliberating a reasonable, yet meaningful, mental health response to an impending potential disaster.

This book examines some of the unique elements of pandemic outbreaks to be considered when formulating a mental health response and explores additional modalities of supplementing and strengthening that response in case of such an outbreak. In addition to focusing on clinical aspects of this issue and associated treatment strategies in addressing it, this text also outlines some public health aspects of planning for mental health responses at various levels (hospital and community), including vaccine hesitancy.

Our daring vision for this book is for it to be an impetus to generating international research and policy interest that would result in steady, serious, and sustained efforts dedicated to understanding this topic. In the interim, we hope that it will serve as a useful starting resource to providers establishing and organizing mental health response in communities afflicted by epidemic or pandemic outbreaks.

References

1. The top 10 causes of death. WHO; 2018 May. https://www.who.int/news-room/fact-sheets/detail/the-top-10-causes-of-death. Accessed Dec 2018.
2. WHO: R&D blueprint, list of blueprint priority diseases. https://www.who.int/blueprint/priority-diseases/en/. Accessed Oct 2018.
3. Strauss S. Ebola research fueled by bioterrorism threat. CMAJ. 2014;186(16):1206. https://doi.org/10.1503/cmaj.109-4910. Epub 2014 Oct 6. PMID: 25288318.
4. Lee BY. Disease X is what may become the biggest infectious threat to our world. Forbes 2018 Mar 10. https://www.forbes.com/sites/brucelee/2018/03/10/disease-x-is-what-may-become-the-biggest-infectious-threat-to-our-world/. Accessed Dec 2018.
5. Emerging pandemic threats, USAID. https://www.usaid.gov/news-information/fact-sheets/emerging-pandemic-threats-program. Accessed Dec 2018.

6. Leeder S. Epidemiology in an age of anger and complaint. Int J Epidemiol. 2017;46(1):1. https://doi.org/10.1093/ije/dyx009.
7. Chan AO, Huak CY. Psychological impact of the 2003 severe acute respiratory syndrome outbreak on health care workers in a medium size regional general hospital in Singapore. Occup Med (Lond). 2004;54(3):190–6. PMID: 15133143.
8. Ofri D. The emotional epidemiology of H1N1 influenza vaccination. N Engl J Med. 2009;361(27):2594–5. https://doi.org/10.1056/NEJMp0911047. Epub 2009 Nov 25. PMID: 19940291.

Chapter 2
Brief History of Pandemics (Pandemics Throughout History)

Damir Huremović

Very few phenomena throughout human history have shaped our societies and cultures the way outbreaks of infectious diseases have; yet, remarkably little attention has been given to these phenomena in behavioral social science and in branches of medicine that are, at least in part, founded in social studies (e.g., psychiatry).

This lack of attention is intriguing, as one of the greatest catastrophes ever, if not the greatest one in the entire history of humankind, was an outbreak of a pandemic [1]. In a long succession throughout history, pandemic outbreaks have decimated societies, determined outcomes of wars, wiped out entire populations, but also, paradoxically, cleared the way for innovations and advances in sciences (including medicine and public health), economy, and political systems [2]. Pandemic outbreaks, or plagues, as they are often referred to, have been closely examined through the lens of humanities in the realm of history, including the history of medicine [3]. In the era of modern humanities, however, fairly little attention has been

D. Huremović (✉)
North Shore University Hospital, Manhasset, NY, USA
e-mail: dhuremov@northwell.edu

© Springer Nature Switzerland AG 2019
D. Huremović (ed.), *Psychiatry of Pandemics*,
https://doi.org/10.1007/978-3-030-15346-5_2

given to ways plagues affected the individual and group psychology of afflicted societies. This includes the unexamined ways pandemic outbreaks might have shaped the specialty of psychiatry; psychoanalysis was gaining recognition as an established treatment within medical community at the time the last great pandemic was making global rounds a century ago.

There is a single word that can serve as a fitting point of departure for our brief journey through the history of pandemics – that word is the *plague*. Stemming from Doric Greek word *plaga* (strike, blow), the word plague is a polyseme, used interchangeably to describe a particular, virulent contagious febrile disease caused by *Yersinia pestis*, as a general term for any epidemic disease causing a high rate of mortality, or more widely, as a metaphor for any sudden outbreak of a disastrous evil or affliction [4]. This term in Greek can refer to any kind of sickness; in Latin, the terms are *plaga* and *pestis* (Fig. 2.1).

Perhaps the best-known examples of plagues ever recorded are those referred to in the religious scriptures that serve as foundations to Abrahamic religions, starting with the Old Testament. Book of Exodus, Chapters 7 through 11, mentions a series of ten plagues to strike the Egyptians before the Israelites, held in captivity by the Pharaoh, the ruler of Egypt, are finally released. Some of those loosely defined plagues are likely occurrences of elements, but at least a few of them are clearly of infectious nature. Lice, diseased livestock, boils, and possible deaths of firstborn likely describe a variety of infectious diseases, zoonoses, and parasitoses [5]. Similar plagues were described and referred to in Islamic tradition in Chapter 7 of the Qur'an (Surat Al-A'raf, v. 133) [6].

Throughout the Biblical context, pandemic outbreaks are the bookends of human existence, considered both a part of nascent human societies, and a part of the very ending of humanity. In the Apocalypse or The Book of Revelation, Chapter 16, seven bowls of God's wrath will be poured on the Earth by angels, again some of the bowls containing plagues likely infectious in nature: "So the first angel went and poured out his bowl on the earth, and harmful and painful sores came upon the people who bore the mark of the beast" (Revelation 16:2).

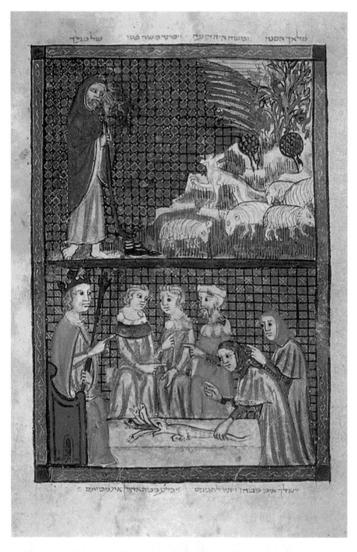

FIGURE 2.1 Plagues of Egypt depicted in Sarajevo Haggadah, Spain, cca. 1350, on display at National Museum of Bosnia-Herzegovina, Sarajevo

Those events, regardless of factual evidence, deeply shaped human history, and continue to be commemorated in religious practices throughout the world. As we will see, the beliefs associated with those fundamental accounts have been rooted in societal responses to pandemics in Western societies and continue to shape public sentiment and perception of current and future outbreaks. Examined through the lens of Abrahamic spiritual context, serious infectious outbreaks can often be interpreted as a "Divine punishment for sins" (of the entire society or its outcast segments) or, in its eschatological iteration, as events heralding the "End of Days" (i.e., the end of the world).

Throughout known, predominantly Western history, there have been recorded processions of pandemics that each shaped our history and our society, inclusive of shaping the very basic principles of modern health sciences. What follows is an outline of major pandemic outbreaks throughout recorded history extending into the twenty-first century.

The Athenian Plague of 430 B.C.

The Athenian plague is a historically documented event that occurred in 430–26 B.C. during the Peloponnesian War, fought between city-states of Athens and Sparta. The historic account of the Athenian plague is provided by Thucydides, who survived the plague himself and described it in his *History of the Peloponnesian War* [7]. The Athenian plague originated in Ethiopia, and from there, it spread throughout Egypt and Greece. Initial symptoms of the plague included headaches, conjunctivitis, a rash covering the body, and fever. The victims would then cough up blood, and suffer from extremely painful stomach cramping, followed by vomiting and attacks of "ineffectual retching" [7]. Infected individuals would generally die by the seventh or eighth day. Those who survived this stage might suffer from partial paralysis, amnesia, or blindness for the rest of their lives. Doctors and other caregivers frequently caught the disease, and died with those whom they had been attempting to heal. The despair caused by the plague within the city led the people to be indifferent to the laws of men and gods, and many cast themselves into self-indulgence [8]. Because of wartime overcrowding in the city of Athens, the plague spread quickly, killing tens of thousands, including Pericles, Athens' beloved leader. With the fall of civic duty and religion, superstition reigned, especially in the recollection of old oracles [7].

The plague of Athens affected a majority of the inhabitants of the overcrowded city-state and claimed lives of more than 25% of the population [9]. The cause of the Athenian plague of 430 B.C. has not been clearly determined, but many diseases, including bubonic plague, have been ruled out as possibilities [10]. While typhoid fever figures prominently as a probable culprit, a recent theory, postulated by Olson and some other epidemiologists and classicists, considers the cause of the Athenian plague to be Ebola virus hemorrhagic fever [11].

The Antonine Plague

While Hippocrates is thought to have been a contemporary of the plague of Athens, even possibly treating the afflicted as a young physician, he had not left known accounts of the outbreak [12]. It was another outbreak that occurred a couple of centuries later that was documented and recorded by contemporary physicians of the time. The outbreak was known as the Antonine Plague of 165–180 AD and the physician documenting it was Galen; this outbreak is also known as the Plague of Galen [13].

The Antonine plague occurred in the Roman Empire during the reign of Marcus Aurelius (161–180 A.D.) and its cause is thought to be smallpox [14]. It was brought into the Empire by soldiers returning from Seleucia, and before it abated, it had affected Asia Minor, Egypt, Greece, and Italy. Unlike the plague of Athens, which affected a geographically limited region, the Antonine plague spread across the vast territory of the entire Roman Empire, because the Empire was an economically and politically integrated, cohesive society occupying wide swaths of the territory [15]. The plague destroyed as much as one-third of the population in some areas, and decimated the Roman army, claiming the life of Marcus Aurelius himself [13].

The impact of the plague on the Roman Empire was severe, weakening its military and economic supremacy. The Antonine plague affected ancient Roman traditions, leading to a renewal of spirituality and religiousness, creating the conditions for spreading of new religions, including Christianity. The Antonine Plague may well have created the conditions for the decline of the Roman Empire and, afterwards, for its fall in the West in the fifth century AD [13].

The Justinian Plague

The Justinian plague was a "real plague" pandemic (i.e., caused by Yersinia Pestis) that originated in mid-sixth century AD either in Ethiopia, moving through Egypt, or in the Central Asian steppes, where it then traveled along the caravan trading routes. From one of these two locations, the pestilence quickly spread throughout the Roman world and beyond. Like most pandemics, the Justinian plague generally followed trading routes providing an "exchange of infections as well as of goods," and therefore, was especially brutal to coastal cities. Military movement at the time also contributed to spreading the disease from Asia Minor to Africa and Italy, and further to Western Europe. Described in detail by Procopius, John of Ephesus, and Evagrius, the Justinian epidemic is the earliest clearly documented example of the actual (bubonic) plague outbreak [16].

During the plague, many victims experienced hallucinations prior to the outbreak of illness. The first symptoms of the plague followed closely behind; they included fever and fatigue. Soon afterwards, buboes appeared in the groin area or armpits, or occasionally beside the ears. From this point, the disease progressed rapidly; infected individuals usually died within days. Infected individuals would enter a delirious, lethargic state, and would not wish to eat or drink. Following this stage, the victims would be "seized by madness," causing great difficulties to those who attempted to care for them [17]. Many people died painfully when their buboes gangrened; others died vomiting blood. There were also cases, however, in which the buboes grew to great size, and then ruptured and suppurated. In such cases, the patient would usually recover, having to live with withered thighs and tongues, classic aftereffects of the plague. Doctors, noticing this trend and not knowing how else to fight the disease, sometimes lanced the buboes of those infected to discover that carbuncles had formed. Those individuals who did survive infection usually had to live with "withered thighs and tongues", the stigmata of survivors. Emperor Justinian contracted the plague himself, but did not succumb [18].

Within a short time, all gravesites were beyond capacity, and the living resorted to throwing the bodies of victims out into the streets or piling them along the seashore to rot. The empire addressed this problem by digging huge pits and collecting the corpses there. Although those pits reportedly held 70,000 corpses each, they soon overflowed [17]. Bodies were then placed inside the towers in the walls, causing a stench pervading the entire city.

Streets were deserted, and all trade was abandoned. Staple foods became scarce and people died of starvation as well as of the disease itself [17]. The Byzantine Empire was a sophisticated society in its time and many of the advanced public policies and institutions that existed at that time were also greatly affected. As the tax base shrank and the economic output decreased, the Empire forced the survivors to shoulder the tax burden [19]. Byzantine army suffered in particular, being unable to fill its ranks and carry out military campaigns, and ultimately failing to retake Rome for the Empire. After the initial outbreak in 541, repetitions of the plague established permanent cycles of infection. By 600, it is possible that the population of the Empire had been reduced by 40%. In the city of Constantinople itself, it is possible that this figure exceeded 50 % [17].

At this point in history, Christian tradition enters the realm of interpreting and understanding the events of this nature [20]. Drawing on the eschatological narrative of the Book of Revelations, plague and other misfortunes are seen and explained as a "punishment for sins," or retribution for the induction of "God's wrath" [21]. This interpretation of the plague will reappear during the Black Death and play a much more central role throughout affected societies in Europe. Meanwhile, as the well-established Byzantine Empire experienced major challenges and weakening of its physical, economic, and cultural infrastructure during this outbreak, the nomadic Arab tribes, moving through sparsely populated areas and practicing a form of protective isolation, were setting a stage for the rapid expansion of Islam [22, 23].

The Black Death

"The Plague" was a global outbreak of bubonic plague that originated in China in 1334, arrived in Europe in 1347, following the Silk Road. Within 50 years of its reign, by 1400, [24] it reduced the global population from 450 million to below 350 million, possibly below 300 million, with the pandemic killing as many as 150 million. Some estimates claim that the Black Death claimed up to 60% of lives in Europe at that time [25].

Starting in China, it spread through central Asia and northern India following the established trading route known as the Silk Road. The plague reached Europe in Sicily in 1347. Within 5 years, it had spread to the virtually entire continent, moving onto Russia and the Middle East. In its first wave, it claimed 25 million lives [24].

The course and symptoms of the bubonic plague were dramatic and terrifying. Boccaccio, one of the many artistic contemporaries of the plague, described it as follows:

> In men and women alike it first betrayed itself by the emergence of certain tumours in the groin or armpits, some of which grew as large as a common apple, others as an egg...From the two said parts of the body this deadly gavocciolo soon began to propagate and spread itself in all directions indifferently; after which the form of the malady began to change, black spots or livid making

their appearance in many cases on the arm or the thigh or elsewhere, now few and large, now minute and numerous. As the
gavocciolo had been and still was an infallible token of approaching death, such also were these spots on whomsoever they showed
themselves [26].

Indeed, the mortality of untreated bubonic plague is close to
70%, usually within 8 days, while the mortality of untreated
pneumonic plague approaches 95%. Treated with antibiotics,
mortality drops to around 11% [27].

At the time, scientific authorities were at a loss regarding
the cause of the affliction. The first official report blamed an
alignment of three planets from 1345 for causing a "great
pestilence in the air" [28]. It was followed by a more generally
accepted miasma theory, an interpretation that blamed bad
air. It was not until the late XIX century that the Black Death
was understood for what it was – a massive Yersinia Pestis
pandemic [29].

This strain of Yersinia tends to infect and overflow the guts
of oriental rat fleas (*Xenopsylla cheopis*) forcing them to
regurgitate concentrated bacteria into the host while feeding.
Such infected hosts then transmit the disease further and can
infect humans – bubonic plague [30]. Humans can transmit
the disease by droplets, leading to pneumonic plague.

The mortality of the Black Death varied between regions,
sometimes skipping sparsely populated rural areas, but then
exacting its toll from the densely populated urban areas, where
population perished in excess of 50, sometimes 60% [31].

In the vacuum of a reasonable explanation for a catastrophe of such proportions, people turned to religion, invoking
patron saints, the Virgin Mary, or joining the processions of
flagellants whipping themselves with nail embedded scourges
and incanting hymns and prayers as they passed from town to
town [32]. The general interpretation in predominantly
Catholic Europe, as in the case of Justinian plague, centered
on the divine "punishment for sins." It then sought to identify
those individuals and groups who were the "gravest sinners
against God," frequently singling out minorities or women.
Jews in Europe were commonly targeted, accused of "poison-
ing the wells" and entire communities persecuted and killed.

Non-Catholic Christians (e.g., Cathars) were also blamed as "heretics" and experienced a similar fate [33]. In other, non-Christian parts of the world affected by the plague, a similar sentiment prevailed. In Cairo, the sultan put in place a law prohibiting women from making public appearances as they may tempt men into sin [34].

For bewildered and terrified societies, the only remedies were inhalation of aromatic vapors from flowers or camphor. Soon, there was a shortage of doctors which led to a proliferation of quacks selling useless cures and amulets and other adornments that claimed to offer magical protection [35].

Entire neighborhoods, sometimes entire towns, were wiped out or settlements abandoned. Crops could not be harvested, traveling and trade became curtailed, and food and manufactured goods became short. The plague broke down the normal divisions between the upper and lower classes and led to the emergence of a new middle class. The shortage of labor in the long run encouraged innovation of labor-saving technologies, leading to higher productivity [2].

The effects of such a large-scale shared experience on the population of Europe influenced all forms of art throughout the period, as evidenced by works by renowned artists, such as Chaucer, Boccaccio, or Petrarch. The deep, lingering wake of the plague is evidenced in the rise of Danse Macabre (Dance of the death) in visual arts and religious scripts [36], its horrors perhaps most chillingly depicted by paintings titled the Triumph of Death (Fig. 2.2) [37].

The plague made several encore rounds through Europe in the following centuries, occasionally decimating towns and entire societies, but never with the same intensity as the Black Death [2].

The Plague Doctor

With the breakdown of societal structure and its infrastructures, many professions, notably that of medical doctors, were severely affected. Many towns throughout Europe

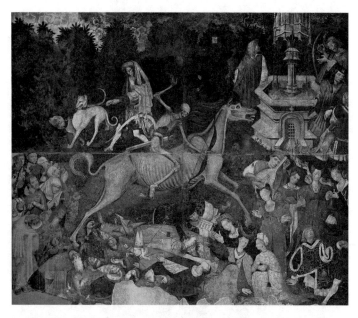

FIGURE 2.2 The Triumph of Death (Trionfo Della Morte), fresco, author unknown, cca. 1446, on display at Palazzo Abatellis, Palermo, Italy

lost their providers to plague or to fear thereof. In order to address this shortage in times of austere need, many municipalities contracted young doctors from whatever ranks were available to perform the duty of the plague doctor (medico della peste) [38]. Venice was among the first city-states to establish dedicated practitioners to deal with the issue of plague in 1348. Their principal task, besides taking care of people with the plague, was to record in public records the deaths due to the plague [39]. In certain European cities like Florence and Perugia, plague doctors were the only ones allowed to perform autopsies to help determine the cause of death and managed to learn a lot about human anatomy. Among the most notable plague doctors of their time were Nostradamus, Paracelsus, and Ambrois Pare [40]. The character of the plague doctor was immortalized by a later invention (from the seventeenth century) of a plague doctor costume by Charles De l'Orme (Fig. 2.3) [41].

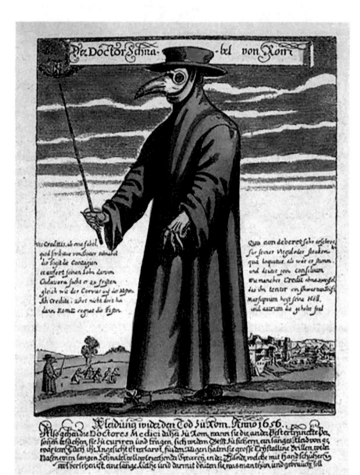

FIGURE 2.3 Doctor Beak (Doctor Schnabel), copper engraving by Paulus Fürst, cca. 1656, from Die Karikatur und Satire in der Medizin: Medico-Kunsthistorische Studie von Professor Dr. Eugen Holländer, 2nd edn (Stuttgart:Ferdinand Enke, 1921), fig. 79 (p. 171)

Quarantine

Drawing from experiences from ancient cultures that had dealt with contagious diseases, medieval societies observed the connection between the passage of time and the eruption of symptoms, noting that, after a period of observation, individuals who had not developed symptoms of the illness would likely not be affected and, more importantly, would not spread the disease upon entering the city. To that end, they started instituting mandatory isolation. The first known quarantine was enacted in Ragusa (City-state of Dubrovnik) in 1377, where all arrivals had to spend 30 days on a nearby island of Lokrum before entering the city. This period of 30 days (trentine) was later extended to 40 days (quarenta giorni or quarantine) [42]. The institution of quarantine was one of the rarely effective measures that took place during the Black Death and its use quickly spread throughout Europe. Quarantine remains in effect in the present time as a highly regulated, nationally and internationally governed public health measure available to combat contagions [43].

"Spanish Flu" Pandemic 1918–1920

The Spanish flu pandemic in the first decades of the twentieth century was the first true global pandemic and the first one that occurred in the setting of modern medicine, with specialties such as infectious diseases and epidemiology studying the nature of the illness and the course of the pandemic as it unfolded. It is also, as of this time, the last true global pandemic with devastating consequences for societies across the globe [44]. It was caused by the H1N1 strain of the influenza virus, [45] a strain that had an encore outbreak in the early years of the twenty-first century.

Despite advances in epidemiology and public health, both at the time and in subsequent decades, the true origin of Spanish flu remains unknown, despite its name. As possible sources of origin, cited are the USA, China, Spain, France, or Austria. These uncertainties are perpetuated by the circumstances of the Spanish flu – it took place in the middle of World War I, with significant censorships in place, and with fairly advanced modes of transportation, including intercontinental travel [44].

Within months, the deadly H1N1 strain of influenza virus had spread to every corner of the world. In addition to Europe, where massive military movements and overcrowding contributed to massive spread, this virus devastated the USA, Asia, Africa, and the Pacific Islands. The mortality rate of Spanish flu ranged between 10% and 20%. With over a quarter of the global population contracting that flu at some point, the death toll was immense – well over 50 million, possibly 100 million dead. It killed more individuals in a year than the Black Death had killed in a century [46].

This pandemic, unusually, tended to mortally affect mostly young and previously healthy individuals. This is likely due to its triggering a cytokine storm, which overwhelms and demolishes the immune system. By August of 1918, the virus had mutated to a much more virulent and deadlier form, returning to kill many of those who avoided it during the first wave [47].

Spanish flu had an immense influence on our civilization. Some authors (Price) even point out that it may have tipped the outcome of World War I, as it affected armies of Germany and the Austrian–Hungarian Empire earlier and more virulently than their Allied opponents (Fig. 2.4) [48].

Many notable politicians, artists, and scientists were either affected by the flu or succumbed to it. Many survived and went on to have distinguished careers in arts and politics (e.g., Walt Disney, Greta Garbo, Raymond Chandler, Franz Kafka, Edward Munch, Franklin Delano Roosevelt, and Woodrow Wilson). Many did not; this pandemic counted as its victims, among others, outstanding painters like Gustav Klimt and Egon Schiele [49], and acclaimed poets like Guillaume Apollinaire. It also claimed the life of Sigmund Freud's fifth child – Sophie Halberstadt-Freud.

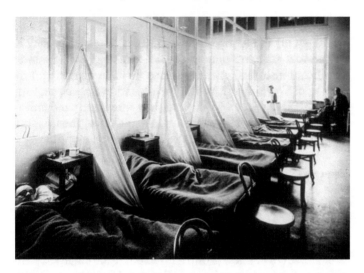

FIGURE 2.4 American Expeditionary Force, victims of Spanish flu in France, 1918. Uncredited U.S. Army photographer – U.S. Army Medical Corps photo via National Museum of Health & Medicine website at U.S. Army Camp Hospital No. 45, Aix-Les-Bains, France, Influenza Ward No. 1

This pandemic was also the first one where the long-lingering effects could be observed and quantified. A study of US census data from 1960 to 1980 found that the children born to women exposed to the pandemic had more physical ailments and a lower lifetime income than those born a few months earlier or later. A 2006 study in the Journal of Political Economy found that "cohorts in utero during the pandemic displayed reduced educational attainment, increased rates of physical disability, lower income, lower socioeconomic status, and higher transfer payments compared with other birth cohorts" [50].

Despite its immense effect on the global civilization, Spanish flu started to fade quickly from the public and scientific attention, establishing a precedent for the future pandemics, and leading some historians (Crosby) to call it the "forgotten pandemic" [51]. One of the explanations for this treatment of the pandemic may lie in the fact that it peaked and waned rapidly, over a period of 9 months before it even could get adequate media coverage. Another reason may be in the fact that the pandemic was overshadowed by more significant historical events, such as the culmination and the ending of World War I. A third explanation may be that this is how societies deal with such rapidly spreading pandemics – at first with great interest, horror, and panic, and then, as soon as they start to subside, with dispassionate disinterest.

HIV Pandemic

HIV/AIDS is a slowly progressing global pandemic cascading through decades of time, different continents, and different populations, bringing new challenges with every new iteration and for every new group it affected. It started in the early 1980s in the USA, causing significant public concern as HIV at the time inevitably progressed to AIDS and ultimately, to death. The initial expansion of HIV was marked by its spread predominantly among the gay population and by high mortality, leading to marked social isolation and stigma.

HIV affects about 40 million people globally (prevalence rate: 0.79%) and has killed almost the same number of people since 1981 [52]. It causes about one million deaths a year worldwide (down from nearly two million in 2005) [53]. While it represents a global public health phenomenon, the HIV epidemic is particularly alarming in some Sub-Saharan African countries (Botswana, Lesotho, and Swaziland), where the prevalence tops 25% [54]. In the USA, about 1.2 million people live with HIV and about 12,000 die every year (down from over 40,000 per year in the late 1990s). HIV in the USA disproportionately affects gay population, transgendered women, and African-Americans [55].

Being a fairly slowly spreading pandemic, HIV has received formidable public health attention, both by national and by international administrations and pharmaceuticals. Advances in treatment (protease inhibitors and anti-retrovirals) have turned HIV into a chronic condition that can be managed by medications. It is a rare infectious disease that has managed to attract the focus of mental health which, in turn, resulted in a solid volume of works on mental health and HIV [56]. By studying the mental health of HIV, we can begin to understand some of the challenges generally associated with infectious diseases. We know, for example, that the lifetime prevalence rate for depression in HIV individuals is, at 22%, more than twice the prevalence rate in general population [57].

We understand how depression in HIV individuals shows association with substance abuse and that issues of stigma, guilt, and shame affect the outlook for HIV patients, including their own adherence to life-saving treatments [58]. We know about medical treatments of depression in HIV and we have studies in psychotherapy for patients with HIV. Some of those approaches can be very useful in treating patients in the context of a pandemic. Given the contrast between the chronicity of the HIV and the acuity of a potential pandemic, most of those approaches cannot be simply translated from mental health approach to HIV and used for patients in a rapidly advancing outbreak or a pandemic.

Smallpox Outbreak in Former Yugoslavia (1972)

Smallpox was a highly contagious disease for which Edward Jenner developed the world's first vaccine in 1798. Caused by the Variola virus, it was a highly contagious disease with prominent skin eruptions (pustules) and mortality of about 30%. It may have been responsible for hundreds of millions of fatalities in the twentieth century alone. Due to the well-coordinated global effort starting in 1967 under the leadership of Donald Henderson, smallpox was eradicated within a decade of undertaking the eradication on a global scale [59].

The smallpox outbreak in the former Yugoslavia in 1972 was a far cry from even an epidemic, let alone a pandemic, but it illustrated the challenges associated with a rapidly spreading, highly contagious illness in a modern world. It started with a pilgrim returning from the Middle East, who developed fever and skin eruptions. Since a case of smallpox had not been seen in the region for over 30 years, physicians failed to correctly diagnose the illness and nine healthcare providers ended among 38 cases infected by the index case and first fatality [60].

Socialist Yugoslavia at the time declared martial law and introduced mandatory revaccination. Entire villages and neighborhoods were cordoned off (cordon sanitaire is a measure of putting entire geographic regions in quarantine). About 10,000 individuals who may have come into contact with the infected were placed in an actual quarantine. Borders were closed, and all non-essential travel was suspended. Within 2 weeks, the entire population of Yugoslavia was revaccinated (about 18 million people at the time). During the outbreak, 175 cases were identified, with 35 fatalities. Due to prompt and massive response, however, the disease was eradicated and the society returned to normal within 2 months [60]. This event has proven to be a useful model for working out scenarios ("Dark Winter") [61] for responses to an outbreak of a highly contagious disease, both as a natural occurrence [62] and as an act of bioterrorism [63].

SARS

Severe Acute Respiratory Syndrome (SARS) was the first outbreak in the twenty-first century that managed to get public attention. Caused by the SARS Corona virus (SARS-CoV), it started in China and affected fewer than 10,000 individuals, mainly in China and Hong Kong, but also in other countries, including 251 cases in Canada (Toronto) [64].

The severity of respiratory symptoms and mortality rate of about 10% caused a global public health concern. Due to the vigilance of public health systems worldwide, the outbreak was contained by mid-2003 [65]. This outbreak was among the first acute outbreaks that had mental health aspects studied in the process and in the aftermath, in various part of the world and in different societies, yielding valuable data on effects of an acute infectious outbreak on affected individuals, families, and the entire communities, including the mental health issues facing healthcare providers [66]. Some of the valuable insights into the mental health of patients in isolation, survivors of the severe illness, or psychological sequelae of working with such patients were researched during the SARS outbreak.

"Swine Flu" or H1N1/09 Pandemic

The 2009 H1N1 pandemic was a reprise of the "Spanish flu" pandemic from 1918, but with far less devastating consequences. Suspected as a re-assortment of bird, swine, and human flu viruses, it was colloquially known as the "swine flu" [67]. It started in Mexico in April of 2009 and reached pandemic proportions within weeks [68]. It began to taper off toward the end of the year and by May of 2010, it was declared over.

It infected over 10% of the global population (lower than expected), with a death toll estimated varying from 20,000 to over 500,000 [69]. Although its death rate was ultimately lower than the regular influenza death rates, at the time it was perceived as very threatening because it disproportionately affected previously healthy young adults, often quickly leading to severe respiratory compromise. A possible explanation for this phenomenon (in addition to the "cytokine storm" applicable to the 1918 H1N1 outbreak) is attributed to older adults having immunity due to a similar H1N1 outbreak in the 1970s [70].

This pandemic also resulted in some valuable data studying and analyzing the mental health aspects of the outbreak. It was among the first outbreaks where policy reports included mental health as an aspect of preparedness and mitigation policy efforts. This outbreak of H1N1 was notable for dissonance between the public sentiment about the outbreak and the public health steps recommended and undertaken by WHO and national health institutions. General public sentiment was that of alarm caused by WHO releases and warnings, but it quickly turned to discontent and mistrust when the initial grim outlook of the outbreak failed to materialize [71]. Health agencies were accused of creating panic ("panicdemic") and peddling unproven vaccines to boost the pharmaceutical companies (in 2009, some extra $1,5 billion worth of H1N1 vaccines were purchased and administered in the USA) [72].

This outbreak illustrated how difficult it may be to gauge and manage public expectations and public sentiments in the effort to mobilize a response. It also demonstrated how distilling descriptions of the impact of a complex public health threat like a pandemic into a single term like "mild," "moderate," or "severe" can potentially be misleading and, ultimately, of little use in public health approach [73].

Ebola Outbreak (2014–2016)

Ebola virus, endemic to Central and West Africa, with fruit bats serving as a likely reservoir, appeared in an outbreak in a remote village in Guinea in December 2013. Spreading mostly within families, it reached Sierra Leone and Liberia, where it managed to generate considerable outbreaks over the following months, with over 28,000 cases and over 11,000 fatalities. A very small number of cases were registered in Nigeria and Mali, but those outbreaks were quickly contained [74]. Ebola outbreak, which happened to be the largest outbreak of Ebola infection to date, gained global notoriety after a passenger from Liberia fell ill and died in Texas in September of 2014, infecting two nurses caring for him, and leading to a significant public concern over a possible Ebola outbreak in the USA [75]. This led to a significant public health and military effort to address the outbreak and help contain it on site (Operation United Assistance) [76, 77].

ZIKA (2015–2016)

Zika virus was a little known, dormant virus found in rhesus monkeys in Uganda. Prior to 2014, the only known outbreak among humans was recorded in Micronesia in 2007. The virus was then identified in Brazil in 2015, after an outbreak of a mild illness causing a flat pinkish rash, bloodshot eyes, fever, joint pain and headaches, resembling dengue. It is a mosquito-borne disease (*Aedes Aegypti*), but it can be sexually transmitted. Despite its mild course, which initially made it unremarkable form the public health perspective, infection with Zika can cause Guillain-Barre syndrome in its wake in adults and, more tragically, cause severe microcephalia in unborn children of infected mothers (a risk of about 1%) [78].

In Brazil, in 2015, for example, there were 2400 birth defects and 29 infant deaths due to suspected Zika infection [79]. Zika outbreak is an illustrative case of the context of global transmission; it was transferred from Micronesia, across the Pacific, to Brazil, whence it continued to spread [78]. It is also a case of a modern media pandemic; it featured prominently in the social media. In early 2016, Zika was being mentioned 50 times a minute in Twitter posts. Social media were used to disseminate information, to educate, or to communicate concerns [80].

Its presence in social media, perhaps for the first time in history, allowed social researchers to study the public sentiment, also known as the emotional epidemiology (Ofri), in real time [81]. While both public health institutions and the general public voiced their concern with the outbreak, scientists and officials sought to provide educational aspect, while concerned public was trying to have their emotional concerns addressed. It is indicative that 4 out of 5 posts on Zika on social media were accurate; yet, those that were "trending" and gaining popularity were posts with inaccurate content (now colloquially referred to as the "fake news") [82]. This is a phenomenon that requires significant attention in preparing for future outbreaks because it may hold a key not only to preparedness, but also to execution of public health plans that may involve quarantine and immunization.

Since 2016, Zika has continued to spread throughout South America, Central America, the Caribbean, and several states within the USA. It remains a significant public health concern, as there is no vaccine and the only reliable way to avoid the risk for the offspring is to avoid areas where Zika was identified or to postpone pregnancy should travel to or living in affected areas be unavoidable [78].

Disease X

Disease X is not, as of yet, an actual disease caused by a known agent, but a speculated source of the next pandemic that could have devastating effects on humanity. Knowing the scope of deleterious effects a pandemic outbreak can have on humankind, in the wake of the Ebola outbreak, the World Health Organization (WHO) decided to dedicate formidable resources to identifying, studying, and combating possible future outbreaks. It does so in the form of an R&D Blueprint, though devising its global strategy and preparedness plan that allows the rapid activation of R&D activities during epidemics [83].

R&D Blueprint maintains and updates a list of so-called identified priority diseases. This list is updated at regular intervals and, as of 2018, it includes diseases such as Ebola and Marburg virus diseases, Lassa fever, Middle East respiratory syndrome coronavirus (MERS-CoV) and Severe Acute Respiratory Syndrome (SARS), Nipah and henipa virus diseases, Zika, and others [84]. For each disease identified, an R&D roadmap is created, followed by target product profiles (i.e., immunizations, treatment, and regulatory framework). Those efforts are important to help us combat a dangerous outbreak of any of the abovementioned diseases, but also to fend off Disease X. Since Disease X is a hypothetical entity, brought by a yet unknown pathogen that could cause a serious international pandemic, the R&D Blueprint explicitly seeks to enable cross-cutting R&D preparedness that is also relevant for both existing culprits and the unknown future "Disease X" as much as possible.

WHO utilizes this R&D Blueprint vehicle to assemble and deploy a broad global coalition of experts who regularly contribute to the Blueprint and who come from several medical, scientific, and regulatory backgrounds. Its advisory group, at the time, does not include mental health specialists [85].

References

1. Benedictow OJ. The black death: the greatest catastrophe ever. Hist Today. 2005;55(3):42–9.
2. Scheidel W. The great leveler: violence and the history of inequality from the stone age to the twenty-first century. Chapter 10: the black death. Princeton: Princeton University Press; 2017. p. 291–313. ISBN 978-0691165028.
3. DeWitte SN. Mortality risk and survival in the aftermath of the medieval black death. PLoS One. 2014;9(5):e96513. https://doi.org/10.1371/journal.pone.0096513.
4. Plague. Merriam-Webster.com. Merriam-Webster, n.d. Web. 2018 Nov 10.
5. Marr JS, Malloy CD. An epidemiologic analysis of the ten plagues of Egypt. Caduceus. 1996;12(1):7–24. PMID: 8673614.
6. The Noble Qur'an Surah 7, v. 133. https://quran.com/7/133.
7. Thucydides, history of the Peloponnesian War, Book 2, Chapter VII. p. 89–100., trans. Crawley R. Digireads.com Publishing; 2017 Sept. ISBN-10: 1420956418.
8. Page DL. Thucydides' description of the great plague. Class Q. 1953;47(3):97–119.
9. Littman RJ. The plague of Athens: epidemiology and paleopathology. Mt Sinai J Med. 2009;76(5):456–67. https://doi.org/10.1002/msj.20137. PMID: 19787658.
10. Langmuir AD, Worthen TD, Solomon J, Ray CG, Petersen E. The Thucydides syndrome: a new hypothesis for the cause of the plague of Athens. N Engl J Med. 1985;313:1027–30.
11. Olson PE, Hames CS, Benenson AS, Genovese EN. The Thucydides syndrome: Ebola Déjà vu? (or Ebola Reemergent?). Emerg Infect Dis. 1996;2(2):155–6. https://doi.org/10.3201/eid0202.960220.
12. Yapijakis C. Hippocrates of Kos, the father of clinical medicine, and Asclepiades of Bithynia, the father of molecular medicine. Review. In Vivo. 2009;23(4):507–14. PMID: 19567383.
13. Sabbatani S, Fiorino S. The Antonine plague and the decline of the Roman empire. Infez Med. 2009;17(4):261–75. Italian. PMID: 20046111.
14. Fears JR. The plague under Marcus Aurelius and the decline and fall of the Roman empire. Infect Dis Clin N Am. 2004;18(1):65–77. PMID: 15081505.
15. Sáez A. The Antonine plague: a global pestilence in the II century d.C. Rev Chil Infectol. 2016;33(2):218–21. https://doi.org/10.4067/S0716-10182016000200011. Spanish. PMID: 27314999.

16. Horgan J. Justinian's Plague (541–542 CE). Ancient history ency-
clopedia; 2014 Dec 26. Retrieved from https://www.ancient.eu/
article/782/

17. Procopius, history of the wars. 7 Vols., trans. Dewing HB, Loeb
Library of the Greek and Roman Classics; 1914. Cambridge, MA:
Harvard University Press. Vol. I, p. 451–73.

18. Rosen W. Justinian's flea: Plague, empire, and the birth of
Europe. New York: Viking Adult, Hardcover; 2007.

19. Smith CA. Plague in the ancient world: a study from Thucydides
to Justinian; 1997. www.loyno.edu/~history/journal/1996-7/Smith.
html

20. Evagrius Scholasticus, Ecclesiastical history (AD431–594), trans.
Walford E; 1846. Book 4. Chapter 29. http://www.tertullian.org/
fathers/evagrius_4_book4.htm#12

21. Evans JAS. The attitude of the secular historians of the age of
Justinian towards the classical past. Traditio. 1976;32:164–5.

22. Sabbatani S, Manfredi R, Fiorino S. The Justinian plague (part
one). Infez Med. 2012;20(2):125–39. Italian. PMID: 22767313.

23. Sabbatani S, Manfredi R, Fiorino S. The Justinian plague (part
two). Influence of the epidemic on the rise of the Islamic empire.
Infez Med. 2012;20(3):217–32. Italian. PMID: 22992565.

24. The Editors of Encyclopaedia Britannica. Black death,
Encyclopædia Britannica; 2018 Sept 4. https://www.britannica.
com/event/Black-Death. Accessed Oct 2018.

25. DeWitte SN. Mortality risk and survival in the aftermath of the
medieval black death. PLoS One. 2014;9(5):e96513. https://doi.
org/10.1371/journal.pone.0096513.

26. Boccaccio, Decameron., trans. Rigg M. London: David Campbell;
1921. Vol. 1, p. 5–11.

27. Centers for Disease Control (CDC). 2015 Sept 24. FAQ: Plague.
https://www.cdc.gov/plague/faq/index.html. Retrieved October
2018

28. Horrox R. Black death. Manchester University Press; 1994.
p. 159. ISBN 978-0-7190-3498-5.

29. Halliday S. Death and miasma in Victorian London: an obstinate
belief. BMJ. 2001;323:1469.

30. Eisen RJ, Gage KL. Adaptive strategies of Yersinia pestis to
persist during inter-epizootic and epizootic periods. Vet Res.
2008;40(2):1.

31. Benedictow OJ. The black death 1346–1353: the complete history. Woodbridge: Boydell Press; 2012. p. 380.

32. Bennett JM, Hollister CW. Medieval Europe: A short history. New York: McGraw-Hill; 2006. p. 326.
33. Gottfried RS. Black death. Simon and Schuster; 2010. p. 74. ISBN 978-1-4391-1846-7.
34. Byrne JP. The black death. Westport: Greenwood Press; 2004. p. 108.
35. Hajar R. The air of history (part II) medicine in the middle ages. Heart Views. 2012;13(4):158–62.
36. Oosterwijk S, Knoell S. Mixed metaphors. The Danse macabre in medieval and early modern Europe. Newcastle upon Tyne: Cambridge Scholars Publishing; 2011. ISBN 978-1-4438-2900-7.
37. Volser I. The theme of death in Italian art: The Triumph of Death [Doctoral dissertation]. McGill University; 2001.
38. Byrne JP. Daily life during the black death. Greenwood Publishing Group; 2006. p. 168–70. ISBN 0-313-33297-5.
39. Wray SK. Communities and crisis: Bologna during the black death. Brill; 2009. p. 172–3. ISBN 978-90-04-17634-8.
40. Hogue J. Nostradamus: the new revelations. Barnes & Noble Books; 1995. p. 1884. ISBN 1-56619-948-4.
41. Boeckl CM. Images of plague and pestilence: iconography and iconology, vol. 27. Kirksville: Truman State University Press; 2000. p. 15.
42. Sehdev PS. The origin of quarantine. Clin Infect Dis. 2002;35(9):1071–2. https://doi.org/10.1086/344062. PMID 12398064.
43. Tognotti E. Lessons from the history of quarantine, from plague to influenza A. Emerging Infectious Diseases. 2013. https://doi.org/10.3201/eid1902.
44. CDC: Remembering the 1918 influenza pandemic. https://www.cdc.gov/features/1918-flu-pandemic/index.html. Accessed Oct 2018.
45. Antonovics J, Hood ME, Baker CH. Molecular virology: was the 1918 flu avian in origin? Nature. 2006;440(7088):E9, discussion E9–10. Bibcode:2006Natur.440E.9A. PMID 16641950. https://doi.org/10.1038/nature04824.
46. Flecknoe D, Charles Wakefield B, Simmons A. Plagues & wars: the 'Spanish flu' pandemic as a lesson from history. Med Confl Surviv. 2018;34(2):61–8. https://doi.org/10.1080/13623699.2018.1472892. Epub 2018 May 15. PMID: 29764189
47. Simonsen L, Clarke MJ, Schonberger LB, Arden NH, Cox NJ, Fukuda K. Pandemic versus epidemic influenza mortality: a

pattern of changing age distribution. J Infect Dis. 1998;178(1):53–60. https://doi.org/10.1086/515616. JSTOR 30114117. PMID 9652423.

48. Price-Smith AT. Contagion and chaos. Cambridge, MA: MIT Press; 2008. ISBN 978-0-262-66203-1.

49. Whitford F. Expressionist portraits. Abbeville Press; 1987. p. 46. ISBN 0-89659-780-6.

50. Almond D. Is the 1918 influenza pandemic over? Long-term effects of in utero influenza exposure in the Post-1940 U.S. population. J Polit Econ. 2006;114(4):672–712. https://doi.org/10.1086/507154.

51. Crosby AW. America's forgotten pandemic: the influenza of 1918. 2nd ed. Cambridge: Cambridge University Press; 2003. ISBN 978-0-521-54175-6.

52. Cohen MS, Hellmann N, Levy JA, DeCock K, Lange J. The spread, treatment, and prevention of HIV-1: evolution of a global pandemic. J Clin Invest. 2008;118(4):1244–54.

53. Wang H, Wolock TM, Carter A, Nguyen G, Kyu H, Gakidou E, Hay SI, Mills EJ, Trickey A. Estimates of global, regional, and national incidence, prevalence, and mortality of HIV, 1980–2015: the global burden of disease study 2015. Lancet HIV. 2016;3(8):e361–87. https://doi.org/10.1016/s2352-3018(16)30087-x. ISSN 2352-3018. PMID 27470028.

54. UNAIDS Data. 2018. http://www.unaids.org/sites/default/files/media_asset/unaids-data-2018_en.pdf

55. Today's HIV/AIDS epidemic factsheet. https://www.cdc.gov/nchhstp/newsroom/docs/factsheets/todaysepidemic-508.pdf. Centers for Disease Control and Prevention. U.S. Government. Accessed Oct 2018.

56. Academy of consultation-Liaison psychiatry, HIV Psychiatry Bibliography. https://www.clpsychiatry.org/member-resources/clinical-monographs/hiv-biblio/. Accessed Oct 2018.

57. Ciesla JA, Roberts JE. Meta-analysis of the relationship between HIV infection and risk for depressive disorders. Am J Psychiatry. 2001;158(5):725–30. PMID: 11329393

58. Safren SA, Bedoya CA, O'Cleirigh C, Biello KB, Pinkston MM, Stein MD, Traeger L, Kojic E, Robbins GK, Lerner JA, Herman DS, Mimiaga MJ, Mayer KH. Cognitive behavioural therapy for adherence and depression in patients with HIV: a three-arm randomised controlled trial. Lancet HIV. 2016;3(11):e529–38. https://doi.org/10.1016/S2352-3018(16)30053-4. Epub 2016 Sep 19. PMID: 27658881.

59. Tarantola D. DA Henderson, Smallpox Eradicator. Am J Public Health. 2016;106(11):1895. PMID: 27715298.
60. Ilic M, Ilic I. The last major outbreak of smallpox (Yugoslavia, 1972): the importance of historical reminders. Travel Med Infect Dis. 2017;17:69–70. https://doi.org/10.1016/j.tmaid.2017.05.010. Epub 2017 May 22. PMID: 28545976.
61. O'Toole T, Mair M, Inglesby TV. Shining light on "dark winter". Clin Infect Dis. 2002;34(7):972–83. Epub 2002 Feb 19. PMID: 11880964.
62. Glasser JW, Foster SO, Millar JD, Lane JM. Evaluating public health responses to reintroduced smallpox via dynamic, socially structured, and spatially distributed metapopulation models. Clin Infect Dis. 2008;46(Suppl 3):S182–94. https://doi.org/10.1086/524382. PMID: 18284358.
63. Nishiura H, Brockmann SO, Eichner M. Extracting key information from historical data to quantify the transmission dynamics of smallpox. Theor Biol Med Model. 2008;5:20. https://doi.org/10.1186/1742-4682-5-20. Review. PMID: 18715509.
64. Smith RD. Responding to global infectious disease outbreaks: lessons from SARS on the role of risk perception, communication and management. Soc Sci Med. 2006;63(12):3113–23. https://doi.org/10.1016/j.socscimed.2006.08.004. PMID 16978751.
65. World Health Organization (WHO). Summary of probable SARS cases with onset of illness from 1 November 2002 to 31 July 2003. http://www.who.int/csr/sars/country/table2004_04_21/en/. Accessed Oct 2018.
66. Maunder RG. Was SARS a mental health catastrophe? Gen Hosp Psychiatry. 2009;31(4):316–7. https://doi.org/10.1016/j.genhosppsych.2009.04.004. Epub 2009 May 22. Review. PMID: 19555790
67. Trifonov V, Khiabanian H, Rabadan R. Geographic dependence, surveillance, and origins of the 2009 influenza A (H1N1) virus. N Engl J Med. 361(2):115–9. https://doi.org/10.1056/NEJMp0904572. PMID 19474418.
68. McNeil Jr DG. In new theory, swine flu started in Asia, not Mexico. The New York Times. 2009 June 23. Accessed Oct 2018.
69. Dawood FS, Iuliano AD, Reed C, et al. Estimated global mortality associated with the first 12 months of 2009 pandemic influenza A H1N1 virus circulation: a modelling study. Lancet Infect Dis. 2012;12(9):687–95. https://doi.org/10.1016/S1473-3099(12)70121-4. PMID 22738893.

70. Nguyen-Van-Tam JS, Openshaw PJM, Hashim A, et al. Risk factors for hospitalisation and poor outcome with pandemic A/H1N1 influenza: United Kingdom first wave (May–September 2009). Thorax. 2010;65(7):645–51. https://doi.org/10.1136/thx.2010.135210. PMC 2921287. PMID 20627925.
71. Garske T, Legrand J, Donnelly CA, Ward H, Cauchemez S, Fraser C, et al. Assessing the severity of the novel influenza A/H1N1 pandemic. BMJ. 2009;339:b2840.
72. Drugmakers, Doctors rake in billions battling H1N1 Flu By Dalia Fahmy. ABC News. 2009 Oct 14. https://abcnews.go.com/Business/big-business-swine-flu/story?id=8820642. Accessed Oct 2018.
73. Leung GM, Nicoll A. Reflections on pandemic (H1N1) 2009 and the international response. PLoS Med. 2010;7(10):e1000346. https://doi.org/10.1371/journal.pmed.1000346.
74. Kalra S, Kelkar D, Galwankar SC, Papadimos TJ, Stawicki SP, Arquilla B, Hoey BA, Sharpe RP, Sabol D, Jahre JA. The emergence of ebola as a global health security threat: from 'lessons learned' to coordinated multilateral containment efforts. J Global Infect Dis. 2014;6(4):164–77.
75. Bell BP, Damon IK, Jernigan DB, et al. Overview, control strategies, and lessons learned in the CDC response to the 2014–2016 Ebola epidemic. Morb Mortal Wkly Rep. 2016;65(3):4–11.
76. CDC: 2014–2016 Ebola outbreak in West Africa. https://www.cdc.gov/vhf/ebola/history/2014-2016-outbreak/. Accessed Oct 2018.
77. Zoroya G. Military Ebola mission in Liberia coming to an end. 2015 Feb 4. https://www.militarytimes.com/2015/02/04/military-ebola-mission-in-liberia-coming-to-an-end/MilitaryTimes. Gannett. Accessed Oct 2018.
78. Kindhauser MK, Allen T, Frank V, Santhanaa RS, Dye C. Zika: the origin and spread of a mosquito-borne virus. Bull World Health Organ. 2016; https://doi.org/10.2471/BLT.16.171082.
79. MFPM A, Souza WV, TVB A, Braga MC, Miranda Filho DB, RAA X, de Melo Filho DA, CAA B, Valongueiro S, APL M, Brandão-Filho SP, CMT M. The microcephaly epidemic and Zika virus: building knowledge in epidemiology. Cad Saude Publica. 2018;34(10):e00069018. https://doi.org/10.1590/0102-311X00069018. English, Portuguese. PMID: 30328996.
80. Wood MJ. Propagating and debunking conspiracy theories on twitter during the 2015-2016 Zika virus outbreak. Cyberpsychol

Behav Soc Netw. 2018;21(8):485–90. https://doi.org/10.1089/cyber.2017.0669. Epub 2018 Jul 18. PMID: 30020821.

81. Ofri D. The emotional epidemiology of H1N1 influenza vaccination. N Engl J Med. 2009;361(27):2594–5. https://doi.org/10.1056/NEJMp0911047. Epub 2009 Nov 25. PMID: 19940291.

82. Sommariva S, Vamos C, Mantzarlis A, Đào LU-L, Tyson DM. Spreading the (fake) news: exploring health messages on social media and the implications for health professionals using a case study. Am J Health Educ. 2018;49(4):246–55. https://doi.org/10.1080/19325037.2018.1473178.

83. WHO: R&D Blueprint, about the R&D Blueprint. https://www.who.int/blueprint/about/en/. Accessed Oct 2018.

84. WHO: R&D Blueprint, list of Blueprint priority diseases. https://www.who.int/blueprint/priority-diseases/en/. Accessed Oct 2018.

85. WHO: R&D Blueprint, scientific advisory group members. https://www.who.int/blueprint/about/sag-members/en/. Accessed Oct 2018.

Chapter 3
Psychology
of the Pandemic

Sameer Khan and Damir Huremović

Mental health of pandemic outbreaks contains parallel processes at two different levels that seem applicable and unique to both concepts of insanity and the concept of plague or contagion.

One process is the mirroring of the pandemic epidemiological process in the realm of psychology – reflecting in thoughts, behaviors, and emotional responses. Just as physical disease has its pathogens, disseminates through vectors, follows the modes of transmission, ferments during the incubation, and erupts to overpower the host, so the public, psychological aspects of the outbreak have kernels of misinformation, feed on uncertainty, grow in doubt as they incubate in the limbic system, and then, through vectors of media and communication, explode in form of individual or mass panic,

S. Khan
Department of Psychiatry, Private Practice, New York, NY, USA

D. Huremović (✉)
North Shore University Hospital, Manhasset, NY, USA
e-mail: dhuremov@northwell.edu

© Springer Nature Switzerland AG 2019
D. Huremović (ed.), *Psychiatry of Pandemics*,
https://doi.org/10.1007/978-3-030-15346-5_3

37

threatening to overpower the coping resources of an individual or an entire community.

The other mirroring process is a parallel between an infectious disease as an actual contagion and mental illness as a symbolic contagion. "Insanity is contagious," writes Joseph Heller in *Catch-22* [1]. We, of course, know that it is not, except our primal instincts are apparently not entirely convinced about that [2].

Hence, the burdensome stigma and isolation of both mental illness and infectious disease, stemming from "fear of contagion." It is, therefore, no wonder that diseases stigmatized in the old days, such as leprosy, became replaced by mental illnesses of the more modern times, sometimes combining into a perfect storm of an infectious pandemic with mental illness and substance abuse on top. Such was the case with HIV, with multiple layers of stigmatization [3].

We ordinarily do not permit those deeply seated fears of contagion and fears of insanity to come to the surface, because the anxieties they generate are intolerable, particularly if they are fused into one. We often, however, indulge in experiencing those terrifying emotions for entertainment purposes. We allow ourselves to be scared by zombies when watching a zombie flick in our state of suspended disbelief because zombies are visibly sick, we know that their sickness is transmissible, and that they could make us sick at any time (unless we get eaten first). At the same time, as a bonus, we are shaken to our core because not only are they physically sick, but because they are also invariably insane and it is the implied loss of our own sanity, our own self, in the process of 'infection' that terrifies us. Zombies that threaten our health and our sanity must, therefore, be removed, banished, or isolated.

The use of zombies in the realm of public health has been lingering since 2003 and *The Zombie Survival Guide* by Max Brooks [4]. It has been a fair game in science since CDC used zombies to illustrate its emergency preparedness segment in 2011 [5]. Zombies have so far been used in numerous campaigns aimed at raising awareness and mounting preparedness for epidemic outbreaks and various other emergencies, from FEMA to mathematicians and pharmacists [6]. Somewhat predictably, after the initial curiosity and amusement with the topic of the "zombie apocalypse," the interest of the target audience begins to wane, leaving no measurable output in its wake [7].

Underlying the dread/fascination with zombies is the ambivalent relationship we have with our own instincts. As early as 1915, Karl Abraham referenced the undead in a letter to Freud, postulating that the oral drive present from the earliest stages of life could lead to the desire to incorporate the loved object by devouring it [8]. This idea had already been taken up by Freud in his *Three Essays on the Theory of Sexuality* [9]. Abraham wondered if such unacceptable cannibalistic urges lead to delusions of being a werewolf or having eaten men or babies – and became the foundations of melancholia over having attacked the object. It was George Romero's *Night of the Living Dead* series that introduced the idea that zombies could be cannibals [8] and this arguably propelled them to capture a greater share of the public imagination. What was being tapped into was the simultaneous identification with the urge to orally attack and incorporate submerged in the *id*, and the horrified disavowal of it – into repulsive zombies that must be exterminated [10].

Common to the generally held beliefs about both zombies and mental illness is the idea of being taken over and losing one's self-determination. Zombies differ from vampires and werewolves, in that they have no volition, they are driven purely by their hunger. They do not have the conscience or the consciousness to have any qualms about their actions [11]. In this, they represent the fantasy of regression to an infantile state where one can feed insatiably without knowledge of one's own aggression [12]. Such regressions occur in both pandemics and in the mass panic associated with them – being invaded, losing control of one's own mind and actions, and being held in the thrall of one's own rapacious hunger and destructive appetite. The end result – a complete giving into one's baser nature leading to the apocalypse and the breakdown of human civilization.

In such a Doomsday, "cast-off resistances, disgust, and anxieties" [13] can be believed to live in the contaminated or infected. These "unfamiliar intruders" (Spillrein, 1995) can then be quarantined in ghettos, attacked, maimed, and killed without compunction. Pandemics include not just the spread of physical illness, but the dissemination of racist, anti-Semitic, homophobic propaganda and pro-violence, limbic agendas that serve to allow our aggressive desires to be simultaneously sated, and projected into the other and destroyed without guilt.

It appears that we indulge these fantasies as a way to simultaneously allow our primal fears and our primitive aggression to come to the fore all in one neat, albeit predictable and repetitive, scenario of a zombie apocalypse. In the same vein, when a potentially dangerous outbreak appears on the horizon, we give in to those impulses again, this time at the collective, societal level. Massive anxiety or massive hysteria heralds and shrouds an actual outbreak and once the outbreak turns out to be contained and subsiding, we turn our heads away and forget about the horrors of anticipating the wave of the pandemic, having conquered our fears [14].

As rational beings and scientists, we appear to be somewhat uncomfortable with the unconscious, primal reactions to possible pandemic outbreaks, so we perhaps choose not to pick them up in our conscious thinking. We can deal with the pandemic as a physical disease, we can deal with the raw, primordial reactions of the public to the outbreak, we can deal with the psychological consequences of those illnesses and outbreaks in the aftermath, but we have a hard time dealing with its dark, charged psychological symbolism within us, right here and now.

A pandemic goes against the widely held conception of a just world ruled by a benevolent higher power; a plague gives lie to the belief of Nature as a nurturing mother or omnipotent God as a nurturing parent. In fact, in the Bible and other religious texts, pandemics were specifically framed as punishments rained down on communities for their sins and infractions. Communities can tolerate sporadic cases of illness amongst individuals within it, but as cases multiply, the ability to absorb the unpredictable, capricious nature of illness over-whelms a community's ability to tolerate uncertainty.

Not only can contagion not be controlled or mastered, but the search for causality creates the unconscious narrative of the pandemic being a result of the community's own badness. Within the community, the well resent and hate the unwell for not only being vectors of illness, but the ostensible reason for the whole community to be damned, expelled from Grace. If zombification separates the soul from the body [15], a pandemic separates a community from its order and its well-being.

The moment order and health are restored, the desire to be seen as good and whole leads to amnesia for the chaos and trauma that preceded recovery. Pandemics disrupt our sense of reality and order, leading to a changed way of storing and metabolizing memories and experiences – and a return to normalcy is accompanied by repression and even amnesia.

This discomfort with acknowledging the deep, existential meaning an outbreak may have for our individual and collec-tive psyche may be reflected in the very first encounter psy-choanalytic theory and practice had with a pandemic. In January 1920, Sophie Freud-Halberstadt, the fifth child of Sigmund Freud, died of complications associated with the Spanish influenza pandemic of 1918–1920. Evidently devas-tated by this loss, Freud writes to Pastor Oskar Pfister: "This afternoon we received the news that our sweet Sophie in Hamburg had been snatched away by influenzal pneumonia, snatched away in the midst of glowing health, from a full and active life as a competent mother and loving wife, all in 4 or 5 days, as though she had never existed. Although we had been worried about her for a couple of days, we had nevertheless been hopeful; it is so difficult to judge from a distance. And this distance must remain distance; we were not able to travel at once, as we had intended, after the first alarming news; there was no train, not even for an emergency. The undis-guised brutality of our time is weighing heavily upon us" [16].

There is a somber, perhaps necessary, almost fatalistic acceptance of the influenza pneumonia evocative of the "com-plete submission to fate" Freud observed among Bosniaks during his 1898 trip to Bosnia-Herzegovina [17]. There is no reflection, no questioning of the grave illness that makes rounds through Europe and takes away young people from the prime of their lives. There is no protest, let alone rage, when travel restrictions due to the flu outbreak prevent him from seeing his dying "Sunday child" or attending her cremation.

In a letter to his friend, Max Eitington Freud writes: "I do not know what more there is to say. It is such a paralyzing event, which can stir no afterthoughts when one is not a believer and so is spared all the conflicts that go with that. Blunt necessity, mute submission" [18]. Visible are grief and devastating loss of a mourning parent, and strikingly absent are critical examinations of the meaning of such events and perhaps the outline of how our self – our id, our ego, our superego perceive and relate to such phenomena. A century later, that silence still persists.

Freud's critical thinking nevertheless may have been affected by this loss as reflected in his next book – *Beyond the Pleasure Principle* (1920) – in which he introduces the concept of death drive. His first biographer, Fritz Wittels, writes: "When Freud made this communication [about death drive] to an attentive world, he was under the impress of the death of the blooming daughter."

Freud himself, however, was not fond of this idea and although he found it "most interesting" in his letter to Wittels, he disavows it: "I should have presumed the existence of a connection between my daughter's death and the train of thought presented in *Beyond the Pleasure Principle*. But the inference that such a sequence exists would have been false" [19].

If death and loss of a loved object is mourned, but not examined, then the agent that caused that death can pass undetected and freely descend back into the depths of the unconscious. Until the next iteration, we are bored and unimpressed by the dormant plagues brewing in the remote parts of the world and of our mind. Boredom here is not an authentic sensation, but merely resistance to a situation where one can be completely overpowered or resulting in significant loss of control [20, 21].

Those of us who deal with the realm of mind in the scientific sense cannot afford to be bored by this subject or to continue to leave it unexamined by being unengaged. Utilizing humor and banality of pop-culture can represent coping styles through which otherwise "boring" and difficult subjects can sometimes be tackled. If that is what it takes, so be it. We can recruit all the zombies of our collective imagination if that will help us better understand the grave psychological implications of a pandemic outbreak and prepare for it. We can venture into the realm of fiction (i.e., science fiction) if that will help us predict the emotional responses and psychological toll of a future outbreak, even if we call it Disease X [22].

The use of zombies and pop culture terminology has permeated other disciplines helping to bolster their efforts to prepare for infectious outbreak disaster scenarios. There is no reason why psychiatry should not do the same, especially since we claim to have the expertise of the realm zombies actually hail from – the depths of our unconscious.

References

1. Heller J. Catch-22: a novel. New York: Simon and Schuster; 1961.
2. Marsh JK, Shanks LL. Thinking you can catch mental illness: how beliefs about membership attainment and category structure influence interactions with mental health category members. Mem Cogn. 2014;42:1011. https://doi.org/10.3758/s13421-014-0427-9.
3. Amerongen DI, Cook LH. Mental illness: a modern-day leprosy? J Christ Nurs. 2010;27(2):86–90.
4. Brooks M. The zombie survival guide, complete protection from the living dead. New York: Penguin Random House; 2003.
5. Preparedness 101: Zombie Apocalypse, Posted on May 16, 2011 by Ali S. Khan, CDC Public Health Matters Blog. https://blogs.cdc.gov/publichealthmatters/2011/05/preparedness-101-zombie-apocalypse/. Accessed July 2018.
6. Baker DE. Pharmacy and the "zombie apocalypse". Hosp Pharm. 2015;50(11):957–8. https://doi.org/10.1310/hpj5011-957.
7. Kruvand M, Bryant FB. Zombie apocalypse: can the undead teach the living how to survive an emergency? Public Health Rep. 2015;130(6):655–63.
8. Abraham K. Letter from Karl Abraham to Sigmund Freud, March 31, 1915. The Complete Correspondence of Sigmund Freud and Karl Abraham 1907–1925, 303–306.

9. Freud S, Strachey J, Richards A. On sexuality: three essays on the theory of sexuality and other works. Harmondsworth: Penguin Books; 1977.

10. Nugent C, Berdine G, Nugent K. The undead in culture and science. Proceedings (Baylor University. Medical Center) 31(2);2018:244–49. PMC. Web. 2018 July 22.

11. Szajnberg NM. Zombies, vampires, werewolves: an adolescent's developmental system for the undead and their ambivalent dependence on the living, and technical implications. Psychoanal Rev. 2012;99(6):897–910.

12. Winnicott DW. The maturational processes and the facilitating environment: studies in the theory of emotional development. New York: International Universities Press; 1965.

13. Rosenfield K. Of zombies, preppers, and bastions: pirates on the Dark Sea of disaster. DIVISION/Rev. 2013;8:9–10.

14. Reconstruction of a Mass Hysteria: The Swine Flu Panic of 2009, Der Spiegel, English Edition. 2010 Mar 12. By Der Spiegel Staff. http://www.spiegel.de/international/world/reconstruction-of-a-mass-hysteria-the-swine-flu-panic-of-2009-a-682613.html

15. Daugherty P. The metaphorical zombie a review of zombie theory: a reader edited by Sarah Juliet Lauro. Death Stud. 2018; https://doi.org/10.1080/07481187.2018.1444928.

16. Halberstadt-Freud, Sophie (1893–1920). International Dictionary of Psychoanalysis. Retrieved July 31, 2018 from Encyclopedia.com: http://www.encyclopedia.com/psychology/dictionaries-thesauruses-pictures-and-press-releases/halberstadt-freud-sophie-1893-1920

17. Freud S, Strachey J. The psychopathology of everyday life. Harmondsworth: Penguin Books; 1975.

18. Rowlinson M. Tennyson's fixations: psychoanalysis and the topics of the early poetry. Charlottesville/London: University Press of Virginia; 1994. p. 165–7.

19. Dufresne T. Tales from the Freudian Crypt: The death drive in text and context. Stanford: Stanford University Press; 2000. p. 29–30.

20. Fenichel O. On the psychology of boredom. In: Rapaport D, editor. Organization and pathology of thought: selected sources. New York: Columbia University Press; 1951. p. 349–61. https://doi.org/10.1037/10584-018.

21. Eastwood JD, Frischen A, Fenske MJ, Smilek D. The unengaged mind: defining boredom in terms of attention. Perspect Psychol Sci. 2012 Sep;7(5):482–95. https://doi.org/10.1177/1745691612456044.

22. Hatchett R. It might sound like science fiction, but disease X is something we must prepare for. The Telegraph. 2018 May 15. https://www.telegraph.co.uk/news/0/must-work-together-prevent-disease-x/

Chapter 4
Societal, Public, and [Emotional] Epidemiological Aspects of a Pandemic

Christy Duan, Howard Linder, and Damir Huremović

The term "contagion" itself has its roots in the Latin word *contagio*, which quite literally means "from touch." Contagion therefore refers to a process of transmission by touch or contact [1]. Contagion theory is a theory of collective behavior that explains how the crowd can cause an impact on individuals' behavior or emotions. The theory is first developed by Gustave Le Bon in his book *The Crowd: A study Of Popular Mind In France* in 1885. In this book, Gustave focused on how a crowd of people could turn the nature of an individual toward the same attitude. He observed that individual behavior would be demoted to the level of the most outspoken person in the crowd. This mass behavior is uncontrollable and

C. Duan (✉)
Department of Psychiatry, Zucker Hillside Hospital, Astoria, NY, USA

H. Linder
Department of Psychiatry, Zucker Hillside Hospital, Glen Oaks, NY, USA

D. Huremović
North Shore University Hospital, Manhasset, NY, USA

© Springer Nature Switzerland AG 2019
D. Huremović (ed.), *Psychiatry of Pandemics*,
https://doi.org/10.1007/978-3-030-15346-5_4

unconscious by the individual. Gustave hypothesized that certain principles must be present for this phenomenon to happen. Firstly, the members of the crowd remain anonymous and are not fearful or anxious about the consequences of the behavior. Secondly, it is the willingness of the individual to sacrifice through collective thinking as a group rather than thinking personally. Lastly, the individual becomes unaware of their behavior and they may engage in behavior in the crowd's behavior [2].

Gustave's theory was later expanded upon by Robert Park and Hubert Blumer. Park's theory argued that people mimic each other's behaviors and emotions when experiencing stress. Blumer contributed to the field of psychological contagion by introducing the term "milling." As described by Blumer, during milling, people become extremely conscious of the crowd's altitudes and respond by adapting these attitudes to avoid external ridicule. A person's independent actions are eliminated through milling which results in displaying of curious behavioral patterns. He concluded his findings with the possibility of the emergence of a new social institution or a social change as the result of this extreme collective behavior. This type of situation could be seen when a large number of people have a specific attitude toward something, it is uncommon that you would find an individual with a differing opinion [3].

Contagion psychology could be subdivided into emotional and behavioral contagions [3, 4].

Emotional contagion is the spread of mood and affect through populations by simple exposures, while behavioral contagion is the propensity for certain behaviors exhibited by one person to be copied by others who are either in the vicinity of the original actor or who have been exposed to media coverage describing the behavior of the original actor [4].

In 1920, William McDougall originally defined emotional contagion as "the principle of direct induction of emotion by way of the primitive sympathetic response." Later psychologists, Elaine Hatfield, John Cacioppo, and Richard Rapson wrote that emotional contagion occurs through automatic mimicry and synchronization of one's expressions, vocalizations, postures, and movements with those of another person. When people unconsciously mirror the crowd's expressions of emotion, they come to feel similar to the overall crowd. Emotional contagion is important to personal relationships because it fosters emotional synchrony between individuals. Emotional contagion happens in a few different stages. The first step occurs when a person imitates another person, for example, if someone waves their hand to say *hello*, you often wave back. Next, a person's emotional experiences could change based on the nonverbal signals of emotions that we give off. For example, a wave of a hand to say *hello* could be a sign of acceptance and acknowledgment, while walking past someone could be a sign of rejection. It has been hypothesized that the limbic system in the brain, mainly the amygdala, allows for emotional attunement and creates the pathway for emotional contagion [4].

In 1979, James Ogunlade defined behavioral contagion as a "spontaneous, unsolicited and uncritical imitation of another's behavior" that occurs when certain variables are met: (a) the observer and the model share a similar situation; (b) the model's behavior encourages the observer to review his condition and to change it as long as the model is seen as a positive influence toward the individual; (c) the model's behavior would assist the observer to resolve a conflict. Behavioral contagion can itself be broken down into six broad areas, based on the nature of the behavior that is spread. They are hysterical contagions, deliberate self-harm contagions, contagions of aggression, rule violation contagions, consumer behavior contagions, and financial contagions [3].

One example of a hysterical contagion was the "June Bug" incident that occurred in a US textile factory in 1962, where 62 factory workers reported having been bitten by a mythical bug that "caused" symptoms such as numbness and nausea. Word of a bug in the factory that would bite its victims and cause them to develop the above symptoms quickly spread. Soon, 62 employees developed this mysterious illness, some of whom were hospitalized. After research by company physicians and experts from the US Public Health Service Communicable Disease Center, it was concluded that the case was one of mass hysteria and that likely stress and anxiety were the cause of the symptoms [5].

There are several factors that determine the rate and extent of behavior and emotional contagion. Some of these are the density and number of the affected community, the personality of the individual, openness to receive and transmit behaviors/feelings, and societal norms membership stability, mood-regulation norms, and task interdependence, and social interdependence. It has been shown that individuals in high-density areas, extroverts rather than introverts, females greater than males, and people with a high degree of identification with the community are more susceptible to social influence.

The notion of contagion theory that individuals do not choose to pass on biological contagions undermines the traditional understanding of the human subject as an autonomous agent. While we may like to believe that individuals consciously and rationally decide on how to respond to situations, social contagion suggests that some of the time, this is simply not the case. Rather than innate human emotion and behaviors, human behaviors/emotions could be thrust upon us from external forces.

Much has been written about the epidemiology of infectious diseases, but the epidemiology of emotions goes neglected. With each outbreak, the rapid spread of disease is heralded by a halo of public panic. Danielle Ofri, MD, Ph.D, introduced this concept of "emotional epidemiology" in a 2009 New England Journal of Medicine perspective. During that year's H1N1 influenza pandemic, Dr. Ofri noted a concurrent emotional pandemic. Her clinic was flooded with desperate calls and anxious walk-in patients demanding answers about H1N1 and the development of the vaccine to prevent it. Six months later, the new vaccine was available. But the panic dissipated just as quickly as it had spread. Her demanding patients were no longer interested in the vaccine. How to explain this dramatic shift in 6 short months? It certainly was not related to logic or facts, since few new medical data became available during this period. She postulated that it reflected a sort of psychological contagion of myth and suspicion [6].

Contagion may be facilitated by many factors, including physical and visual proximity in the setting of dramatic situations or occurrences. New viruses that have never been seen before, initially often without a recognized cure, could cause widespread fear and panic. In particular, the drama engendered by emergency response teams coupled with eager newscasters can lend credence to false beliefs that something serious has occurred, and it can fuel what is perhaps the real disease agent in many cases of mass hysteria: anxiety. This anxiety could also be propagated through social media, often causing the anxiety itself "to go viral." Sensationalism has long been recognized as a successful strategy to sell newspapers and news outlets may exaggerate the importance of unusual medical cases. In a poll of 2256 adults commissioned by the National Health Council, medical and health news stories in the media were powerful influences, causing more than half of viewers and readers to take some action regarding their health [7].

In epidemiology, mathematical models are used to study how infectious diseases spread, understand the course of illness, predict outbreak patterns, and identify strategies to control the disease. John Graunt was the first to analyze causes of death in his 1662 book, *Natural and Political Observations Made Upon the Bills of Mortality*. At the time, weekly statistics of death were called *bills of mortality* and published by London officials to monitor the bubonic plague [8, 9].

Since then, epidemiologic models and surveillance have matured significantly. Perhaps the most important recent technological advance is the internet [9]. Leveraging social media for real-time reporting of infectious disease has been identified as one way to create an efficient public surveillance system for early detection and immediate response. Utilizing and disseminating facts and solid evidence in cases of an outbreak by relying on dependable public health and epidemiological data is perhaps the best way of countering the anxiety-inducing uncertainties, rumors, and speculations [10].

We need, however, to learn much more about how to address a possible emotional pandemic accompanying an actual outbreak. There are several transnational, national, and private agencies that are able to run complex models of an outbreak, accounting for many variables [11]. There is, however, a lack of studies and models that can predict mass psychological reactions and behaviors in rapidly spreading outbreaks. Creating these models is crucial for managing outbreaks. Fear thrives on ignorance and misinformation can be, spontaneously or deliberately, used to manipulate emotional responses [10]. In case of an outbreak, fear and ignorance can lead to panic and uncontrollable behaviors on a massive scale that may have deleterious effects for entire societies.

If an epidemic or pandemic outbreak is intentionally triggered, in case of bioterrorism or biological warfare, then the very aspect of emotional epidemiology and public emotional response itself becomes a target and a battlefield in the age of modern communication and social media. A crisis of significant proportions with considerable risks and a great number of unknown variables generates a tremendous public demand for information and that demand is likely to be a suitable target for malicious feeds containing rumors, half-truths, and "fake news" [12]. This informational challenge is potentially augmented by other components of a pandemic that generate strong public emotional and attitudinal reactions, such as social distancing (quarantine) and immunization. Any organized hostile activity accompanying an intentional outbreak will likely seek to maximize impact by heavily manipulating the pre-existing and the developing public attitudes toward mandated measures aiming at curtailing the outbreak.

Knowing all this, mental health professionals should embrace their interdisciplinary role as both consultants and as a liaison between epidemiologists, public health officials, and the general public. Familiarizing themselves with basic epidemiological concepts will allow mental health professionals to understand the emotional impact of outbreaks and provide useful recommendations. For example, the length of incubation of an infectious pathogen could determine the recommended duration of quarantine, which is known to have a significant emotional impact on quarantined individuals. This chapter includes a glossary of terms that will allow mental health professionals to converse competently with infectious disease colleagues, and also help relay that information to the general public.

Glossary [13, 14]

Case	a person with a disease
Primary case	the initial person infected with a disease, sometimes referred to as the index case or patient zero
Secondary case	a person infected by the primary case
Basic reproduction number (R_0, r *nought*)	the number of secondary cases produced by a single infection in a previously unaffected population. This number depends on how long a person is infectious, how infectious the disease is, and the contact between the infected person and the susceptible population. In general, if $R_0 < 1$, the infection will die out in the long run but if $R_0 > 1$, the infection will be able to spread in a population. The larger the value of R_0, the more contagious the illness and the harder it gets to control the epidemic.
Case fatality rate	the proportion of deaths among cases over the disease course. It can be expressed as a percentage.
Epidemic	the rapid spread of an infectious disease to a large number of people in a population

Incidence rate	the proportion of newly diagnosed cases among unaffected people at risk for the disease over a given period of time
Incubation, or latency period	the length of time between exposure to an infected person and acquiring an infection until symptoms emerge
Infectivity	the ability of a disease agent to establish an infection
Morbidity	having a disease
Co-morbidity	having more than one disease simultaneously
Mortality	the proportion of deaths due to a disease among the total population over a period of time (not to be confused with case fatality rate)
Lead time	the length of time between the early detection of a disease through screening and its usual diagnosis based on clinical presentation
Outbreak	the rapid increase of a disease in a population
Pandemic	a large epidemic that affects several countries or continents
Prevalence rate	the proportion of total number of cases among the entire population at any given time
Time course	the typical stages of illness of an infectious disease
Transmission	the spread of an infectious disease from the infected to the uninfected

For those interested in more basics on epidemiology, CDC maintains several courses on principles of epidemiology in public health practice [14].

References

1. Marsden P. Memetics & social contagion: two sides of the same coin? J Memet Evol Model Inf Transm. 1998;2:171–85.
2. Stephenson GM, Fielding GT. An experimental study of the contagion of leaving behavior in small gatherings. J Soc Psychol. 1971;84(1):81–91.
3. Wheeler L. Toward a theory of behavioral contagion. Psychol Rev. 1966;73(2):179–92. https://doi.org/10.1037/h0023023.
4. Hatfield E, Cacioppo JT, Rapson RL. Emotional contagion. Curr Dir Psychol Sci. June 1993;2(3):96–9.
5. Kerckhoff AC, Back KW. The June Bug: a study of hysterical contagion. New York: Appleton-Century-Crofts; 1968.
6. Ofri D. The emotional epidemiology of H1N1 influenza vaccination. N Engl J Med. 2009;36(27):2594–5.
7. Johnson T. Medicine and the media. New Engl J Med. 1998;339(2):87–92.
8. Graunt J. Natural and political. 5th ed. London: John Martyn\ Royal Society.
9. Morabia A. Epidemiology's 350th anniversary: 1662–2012. Epidimiology. 2013;24(2):179–83.
10. Wood MJ. Propagating and debunking conspiracy theories on twitter during the 2015–2016 Zika virus outbreak. Cyberpsychol Behav Soc Netw. 2018;21(8):485–90. https://doi.org/10.1089/cyber.2017.0669. Epub 2018 Jul 18. PMID: 30020821.
11. The Institute for Disease Modeling. http://www.idmod.org/home. Accessed Oct 2018.
12. Sommariva S, Vamos C, Mantzarlis A, Đào LU-L, Tyson DM. Spreading the (fake) news: exploring health messages on social media and the implications for health professionals using a case study. Am J Health Educ. 2018;49(4):246–55. https://doi.org/10.1080/19325037.2018.1473178.
13. Principles of epidemiology in public health practice, third edition an introduction to applied epidemiology and biostatistics, lesson 1: introduction to epidemiology. https://www.cdc.gov/ophss/csels/dsepd/ss1978/lesson1/index.html. Accessed Oct 2018.
14. CDC: principles of epidemiology in public health practice, third edition an introduction to applied epidemiology and biostatistics. https://www.cdc.gov/ophss/csels/dsepd/ss1978/. Accessed Oct 2018.

Chapter 5
The Importance of Culture in Managing Mental Health Response to Pandemics

Guitelle St. Victor and Saeed Ahmed

Introduction

In recent years, the world has witnessed a number of epidemic outbreaks with devastating effects. While outbreaks are inevitable, their impact can be mitigated. Effective management of such events calls for better approaches encompassing all the different aspects that can influence the outcome, including the cultural aspect. Communities' response to outbreaks and their willingness to embrace the interventions devised and implemented by international experts in order to mitigate the effects of an outbreak can greatly influence the outcome [11]. There have been considerable challenges with managing outbreaks in some parts of Africa due to the strong influence of traditional beliefs on the response to the outbreaks and to the measures instituted to

G. St. Victor (✉) · S. Ahmed
Department of Psychiatry, Nassau University Medical Center, East Meadow, NY, USA

© Springer Nature Switzerland AG 2019   55
D. Huremović (ed.), *Psychiatry of Pandemics*,
https://doi.org/10.1007/978-3-030-15346-5_5

counter them. The outbreak of the Zika virus, similarly, presented unanticipated healthcare challenges. The case of the Ebola pandemic in West Africa can help develop a deeper insight into the issue of pandemics and the cultural response observed and its effect on the outcome of the event.

A Brief Literature Review

Agusto, Teboh-Ewungkem, and Gumel [2] examine the effect of customs and traditional beliefs on the transmission dynamics of Ebola outbreaks. The authors argued that in the early stages of the Ebola pandemic in Africa, cultural beliefs played an important role that contributed to the spreading of the disease. They suggest that an identification of the crucial cultural parameters of the epidemic is vital to the development of an efficient control strategy. Similarly, Manguvo and Mafuvadze [10] also ponder the essential role of culture in the Ebola epidemic in African countries. The authors highlighted other social factors that were also responsible for the spread of Ebola, such as a general lack of awareness and the poor state of health facilities. Embracing of specific religious and cultural practices by some of the West African communities are also found to have an adverse impact on the outbreak. For example, there is a common belief that outbreaks are a consequence of transgressions against God and for which God strikes people with diseases. Some maintain that the Ebola outbreak is God's punishment for indulgence in adultery and homosexuality [17]. Even when interventions to combat the outbreak were being deployed, some of the West African communities could not readily accept all science-based intervention due to the prevailing belief that the disease was a punishment from the ancestral spirits or God for various transgressions such as breaking taboos [10]. As for the healing process in the aftermath, a good proportion of the members of the community believed strongly in traditional and spiritual healing, a factor that served to complicate the situation further. Prevailing cultural beliefs sometimes represent a challenge for healthcare providers (often international aid workers) in communicating the causes and nature of epidemics such as Ebola to local communities in a meaningful way. Even though modern medicine has become the healthcare norm throughout Africa, there is also still a heavy reliance on traditional medical practices among many African communities. Traditional healers may fail to understand that Ebola is a viral infection with the potential of causing numerous deaths within a short time [7]. The inadequate understanding of the epidemic leads to further complications, such as unsafe handling of remains that become a source of contamination of the water supply by unburied dead bodies, or burial practices, which propagate the illness. Like all communities, African communities tend to have specific burial rituals that must be adhered to when laying their loved ones to rest [3]. During the period of epidemic disasters, it becomes challenging for health professionals and researchers to investigate dead bodies because affected communities tend to bury their loved ones according to their burial rituals, which makes it difficult to determine the cause of death or to approximate the risks to the rest of the population.

Evidence-based public health methods are preferred to combat outbreaks of a highly infectious disease such as Ebola, but because of the critical role of traditional and cultural factors that play in addressing these outbreaks, a holistic approach must be considered in order to meaningfully influence the outcome [9]. Failing to incorporate cultural and contextual factors may limit the degree of success in controlling the spread of diseases. Simultaneously, during the outbreaks, it can be noted that there is an initial resistance to the evidence-based approaches to limiting the spread of Ebola in some of the affected communities [10]. Therefore, the best approach to promote health in such disasters lies in understanding and, to a reasonable degree, embracing both traditional and religious practices. A recently published study shows that traditional and cultural beliefs can significantly contribute to the challenges that the health practitioners had in managing the outbreak [2].

The longer lasting psychological consequences tend to manifest after the crisis [8] and the case of Ebola was not any different from other disasters. Mental health care after such an outbreak remains a challenge throughout the region, with or without international aid. For example, the World Health Organization (WHO) implemented a mental health capacity building program for Ebola survivors [5]. The program initially showed positive results, but a disruption in funding for the project adversely impacted the supervision and follow-up training and rolled back the initial gains. The differences in the traditional cultures from country to country may have a role to play in the instability in that particular region, for example, Guinea's cultures are rich in oral histories, the supernatural powers, dreams, and contracts with ancestral spirits. The people trust their elders, seeing them as the custodians of culture. They also depend on traditional healers and the Griots (storytellers) who guide them regarding the rules by which they live [5]. The emergence of the Ebola virus disease (EVD) epidemic appeared to reinvigorate cultural practices that were fading with time. A renewed interest in the revival of indigenous knowledge and traditions ensures that these get properly transmitted from one generation to the next. The revival efforts represent a direct attempt to establish connections with the community, the ancestors, and the past, serving to reinstate social order. Past studies show that such cultural preservation may constitute a protective factor in mental and physical health and promote social cohesion. Efforts to preserve the indigenous culture may result in a higher quality of life and improved health and sense of well-being. The previous studies and past experiences show a promise in managing adverse effects in the aftermath of an EVD epidemic, as was the case in Guinea. Programs creating professional and institutional opportunities to promote diversity of cultural expression, support cultural preservation and traditional rituals can serve as catalysts for the restoration of communities in grief after the devastation from EVD [5].

Tucci, Moukaddam, Meadows [13] reported that mental health issues that occur with epidemics and emerging diseases are rarely examined and even sometimes deliberately ignored due to cultural considerations. The available literature on outbreaks lacks sufficient evidence to determine a relationship between an epidemic such as EVD and mental illness, yet there is a considerable need for psychiatric care in the wake of such an outbreak [13]. Patients in such circumstances tend to experience symptoms of major depressive disorder (MDD), post-traumatic stress disorder (*PTSD*), and even suicidal ideations. Those combating epidemics through public health projects, therefore, need to advocate for more extensive research on mental health in such circumstances. There is also a need to enhance public awareness of the neuropsychiatric complications evolving from these outbreaks and offer the appropriate treatment and support, wherever necessary, and culturally appropriate, and whenever possible.

Epidemics of the developing world differ from epidemics of the developed countries, both in causing agents and in their proportions. Epidemics are a part of daily life in many developing countries, often accompanying poverty, civil unrest, armed conflicts, or natural disasters. Among many current pandemics, one of the most dangerous ones was a severe dengue epidemic, with massive dengue outbreaks occurring in 2016. The Americas reported more than 2.38 million cases in 2016, with Brazil alone recording slightly less than 1.5 million cases (WHO Fact Sheet/Dengue and severe dengue 2018). In 2018, dengue was also reported in Bangladesh, Cambodia, India, Myanmar, Malaysia Pakistan, Philippines, Thailand, and Yemen. Similarly, *cholera outbreaks* have been making rounds for the past 200 years. A total of three to five million cases of cholera occur worldwide annually, and 100,000 to 120,000 of these result in death (WHO [16] Report on Cholera). The spread of cholera is greatly facilitated by fecal contamination of water supplies and a lack of treatment of the drinking water. Outbreaks of cholera killed millions of lives from time to time in many regions of the world. Between 1817 and 1860, deaths from a cholera outbreak in India are estimated to have exceeded 15 million people. Another 23 million died between 1865 and 1917, during the next three outbreaks. In recent times, the world witnessed another cholera outbreak 10 months after the January 2010 earthquake in Haiti. This outbreak that killed at least 10,000 people may have actually been brought on by those who came to Haiti to help a community in distress – UN workers. This unfortunate chain of events caused considerable stress and tension in the affected communities and negatively impacted the public health response to the outbreak [6]. Some local communities suspected even that cholera was being deliberately spread by international agencies, or that it was related to religious aspects such as voodoo practices. In response to such attitudes, the Haitian Red Cross initiated several activities with a psychosocial component, emphasizing respect for Haitian people's perceptions and beliefs. This endeavor demonstrated that building trust with the affected community during an outbreak is the key to deliver an effective message. Experiences from responders show that psychosocial support interventions may play a critical role in response to such epidemics.

Addressing the Challenges of Religious and Cultural Practices

Implementing effective management options during outbreaks to address health and safety concerns may be a challenge in some cultural paradigms. Burial practices for the deceased turned out to be one the most important modes of spreading the disease – a common ritual among many religions is washing the dead body with bare hands and spending time with the dead body, which, in the case of Ebola, may be highly contagious. In the case of Muslims who succumbed to EVD, their deceased bodies were covered in white bags as opposed to the traditional white cotton [4]. In this and other cultures, burial workers would attempt to honor requests from the families of the deceased that they found acceptable and safe. For instance, burial workers who dressed in protective suits would dress the dead in outfits of the family's choice before placing them in body bags. Jewelry, money, and other items considered to be of sentimental value to the deceased would also be included in the body bags [4].

Some countries and governments demonstrated formidable vigilance regarding the psychosocial aspects of the EVD outbreak. The government of Ghana, for example, set up an inter-ministerial committee to lead a preparation and containment plan, although the country managed to avoid an EVD outbreak altogether. The committee collaborated with the country's development partners to establish a preparedness and response plan at the national level. The country's Health Service conducted intensive risk communication and social mobilization countrywide as part of the EVD response plan [1]. There was also the constitution of EVD response teams at the national, regional, and district levels. The government's efforts aimed at mitigating an EVD outbreak due to cross-border travels to and from countries affected by the crisis. Given the impact of certain cultural factors and spread of the infection, the Ghanaian government was keen on exploring the influence of those factors in its prevention, also on preparing its population better in case of an outbreak [1].

Prevention Strategies for the Rest of the World

During the Ebola outbreak in West Africa, there was a notable delay in international assistance blamed due to the absence of leadership and coordinated response [12]. Various international organizations can come up with strategies to address the challenges presented by cultural and religious practices in the handling of an Ebola crisis. Some of them have already stepped up their efforts in this direction in order to enhance positive outcomes. UNESCO's efforts for instance in addressing the EVD crisis have been prominent at the global level [14]. UNESCO's expertise comes from their knowledge of different cultures and various educational systems. Furthermore, the close working relationship that they enjoy with other entities such as health ministries, United Nations agencies, and civil societies also help them to prepare a better response environment. The organization has also learned from its vast experience in handling HIV-related issues that education alone without close attention to cultural factors is insufficient in addressing the cultural and social factors that impact efforts to mitigate or manage an outbreak [14].

WHO (World Health Organization) has, on its part, provided leadership in addressing the Ebola outbreak in areas where communities cultural practices appeared to be incompatible with scientific approaches to control the outbreak. The organization has developed a managerial framework for Ebola and its plan ensures that the organization has a fully staffed emergency response team in place in different countries [15]. WHO has an extra capacity of human resources to be sent to areas that are in greater need of its services such as those currently experiencing outbreaks. The organization's response plan builds on its past experiences with pandemics and its strategies have proven to be successful. Getting the transmission rates down to zero implies that in addition to the therapeutic approaches, WHO staff will work within the context of cultural practices and beliefs of the affected community [15]. Culture cannot be ignored, as it tends to find its way back into any organized public health project. As such, much can be gained by embracing it instead of rejecting it or ignoring it, and that inclusion was one of the guiding principles behind WHO's protocol on safe and dignified burials [15].

Conclusion

Local cultural and religious framework affect the outcome of international interventions aimed at containing pandemics as was the case with the Ebola crisis in West Africa in 2014–2015. Certain religious and cultural practices can have an adverse impact by serving as modes of transmission. Some beliefs, attitudes, and practices also impact the mental health of the survivors in the aftermath of the crisis. It is, therefore, challenging to design and implement universal approaches without adjusting them so that local communities can effectively embrace the management of the outbreak. One should always look for adaptations that can be implemented by the affected communities, which will effectively address health and safety concerns, while respecting prevalent cultural norms. International aid agencies, unfortunately, often tend to look at an epidemic through a public health hazard lens, without understanding the cultural aspects embedded in it. More deliberate efforts, however, by various international stakeholders to incorporate cultural and religious aspects in their response can go a long way in ensuring optimal outcome of extinguishing an outbreak.

Acknowledgement The Authors sincerely thank Tayo Akadiri, MS III, for the research on this chapter.

References

1. Adongo PB, Tabong PTN, Asampong E, Ansong J, Robalo M, Adanu RM. Preparing towards preventing and containing an Ebola virus disease outbreak: what socio-cultural practices may affect containment efforts in Ghana? PLoS Negl Trop Dis. 2016;10(7):e0004852.
2. Agusto FB, Teboh-Ewungkem MI, Gumel AB. Mathematical assessment of the effect of traditional beliefs and customs on the transmission dynamics of the 2014 Ebola outbreaks. BMC Med. 2015;13(1):96.
3. BMC. When culture meets epidemic: the case of Ebola – On Medicine. 2015 Apr 23. Retrieved from https://blogs.biomedcentral.com/on-medicine/2015/04/23/culture-ebola/
4. Coltart CE, Lindsey B, Ghinai I, Johnson AM, Heymann DL. The Ebola outbreak, 2013–2016: old lessons for new epidemics. Phil Trans R Soc B. 2017;372(1721):20160297.
5. Faregh N, Kemo S, Tounkara A. Rethinking the role of culture in mental health after the Ebola epidemic | The Lancet Global Health Blog. 2016 Nov 4. Retrieved September 1, 2018, from http://globalhealth.thelancet.com/2016/11/04/rethinking-role-culture-mental-health-after-ebola-epidemic
6. Grimaud J, Legagneur F. Community beliefs during a cholera outbreak intervention. 2011;9(1):26–34.
7. Hewlett BS, Hewlett BL. Ebola, culture, and politics: the anthropology of an emerging disease. Belmont: Cengage Learning; 2007.

8. IASC. Mental health and psychosocial support in Ebola virus disease outbreaks. 2015. Retrieved September 1, 2018, from http://www.who.int/mental_health/emergencies/ebola_guide_for_planners.pdf

9. Li V. Ebola, emerging: the limitations of culturalist discourses in epidemiology. J Glob Health. 2014. http://www.ghjournal.org/ebola-emerging-the-limitations-of-culturalist-discourses-in-epidemiology/.

10. Manguvo A, Mafuvadze B. The impact of traditional and religious practices on the spread of Ebola in West Africa: time for a strategic shift. Pan Afr Med J. 2015;22(Suppl 1):9.

11. Peters A. The importance of culture in managing epidemics: what Ebola can teach us about Zika – GCSP. 2016 Feb 10. Retrieved August 30, 2018, from https://www.gcsp.ch/News-Knowledge/Global-insight/The-Importance-of-Culture-in-Managing-Epidemics-What-Ebola-can- teach-us-about-Zika

12. Southall HG, DeYoung SE, Harris CA. Lack of cultural competency in international aid responses: the Ebola outbreak in Liberia. Front Public Health. 2017;5:5.

13. Tucci V, Moukaddam N, Meadows J, Shah S, Galwankar SC, Kapur GB. The forgotten plague: psychiatric manifestations of Ebola, zika, and emerging infectious diseases. J Global Infect Dis. 2017;9(4):151.

14. UNESCO. UNESCO's responseto Ebola: strategy paper. 2014. Retrieved from https://www.google.com/url?sa=t&rct=j&q=&esrc=s&source=web&cd=7&cad=rja&uact

15. WHO. Ebola response: what needs to happen in 2015. 2015. Retrieved August 30, 2018, from http://www.who.int/csr/disease/ebola/one-year-report/response-in-2015/en/

16. World Health Organization. Cholera. Geneva: World Health Organzation, Media Centre; 2012 Jul. Fact sheet no. 107; http://www.who.int/mediacentre/factsheets/fs107/en. [Context Link]. http://www.who.int/news-room/fact-sheets/detail/dengue-and-severe-dengue

17. World Health Organization: African traditional medicine day. 2010. http://ahm.afro.who.int/special-issue14/ahm-special-issue-14.pdf.

Chapter 6
Preparing for the Outbreak

Damir Huremović

An approaching outbreak requires planning at the institutional and community level. Every healthcare facility is a potential nexus of particular stress because facilities are the locales where patients with an active infection will congregate and seek help. This burden of patient influx puts a dual stressor on the staff – one is possible mandatory overtime to the extent of shelter-in-place and isolation scenarios, and the other is the very possibility of contracting the infection and succumbing to it.

Preparations are important particularly for the existing population of mental health patients. One set of preparations should be put in place for patients in the community, the other for residential patients and patients housed at mental health facilities.

Mental health patients who are in the community are at risk for developing more anxiety about the arriving pandemic, particularly if they are already treated for anxiety

D. Huremović (✉)
North Shore University Hospital, Manhasset, NY, USA
e-mail: dhuremov@northwell.edu

© Springer Nature Switzerland AG 2019   65
D. Huremović (ed.), *Psychiatry of Pandemics*,
https://doi.org/10.1007/978-3-030-15346-5_6

spectrum disorders. Worrying about pandemic can lead to a worsening of existing mood disorders, such as depression.

One chart review study from the 2009 H1N1 influenza outbreak revealed that children receiving mental health care and patients with neurotic and somatoform disorders may be particularly vulnerable to psychological effects of infectious disease epidemics [1].

Patients who are seriously mentally ill and who are particularly concerned about the consequences of the outbreak may break with their compliance and risk relapses of serious mental illnesses such as schizophrenia, schizoaffective disorder, or bipolar disorder. Patients may demonstrate impairment of judgment, become reckless and engage in risk-taking behaviors. The risk of such behaviors may be accentuated in the context of an outbreak.

Because of reckless behavior associated with impaired judgment or because of poor self-care due to the chronicity of their illness, mental health patients may have difficulties following general public instructions and orders and put themselves at risk for violating various measures aimed at mitigating the outbreak.

It is conceivable that during and after an outbreak, communications and transportation may be disrupted. Access to mental health care in the community under such circumstances may become impossible. It pays to foresee the need for medications for a discrete period of time for a given population and make sure those medications are dispatched to forward points of care in advance. Alternately, medications can be given to patients and their families for more than a month in advance, but this ought to be weighed about potential risks for overdose and abuse.

Medications that require strict monitoring (lithium, clozapine) can be converted to other medications, if feasible. If not, levels should be obtained as close to the arrival of an outbreak and again as soon as possible afterwards. An alternate, if untried, approach would be to obtain stable levels within normal parameters at a certain dose and then lower the dose somewhat should the lack of access continue and should lab work remain unavailable.

Even if medications are distributed in advance and available, patients may still not be able to reach their providers for regular care. The use of telecommunications, if available and not disrupted, may be of paramount importance, as it can ensure the continuity of care, including assessment and psychotherapy. Because of the specific needs of this population, tele-mental health checks can also be used to provide mental status and compliance monitoring, general health information, and other assistance.

For patients with substance abuse problems, particularly those on maintenance therapies, uninterrupted delivery of medications could create a significant problem. Some of the options include detoxification prior to the arrival of an outbreak or stockpiling medications with patients for prolonged use; each coming with its own set of risks and complications.

Some alternate approaches which could be considered include providing automatic dispensaries (similar to ATMs, only for medications), an option dependent on electricity supply, delivering medications with unmanned aerial vehicles (drones), or storing limited quantities of medication at different locations, each for a limited period of time, to be disclosed to patients at certain intervals. These options, again, depend on the existence and functioning of telecommunications infrastructure in the affected area [2].

In residential facilities, the situation is complicated by a congregation of a number of individuals at one place. Little evidence exists on how to prepare for an outbreak at the residential level. A report from H1N1 planning at a residential facility in New Zealand indicated that key lessons learned were: planning and managing for infectious diseases should be part of disaster planning, knowing clients and community, sharing knowledge and information, supporting the mental health of individuals throughout – including the staff, and expecting reactions as part of recovery [3].

The challenges of caring for a number of individuals in a mental hospital or a residential facility are fairly evident. It is no wonder that about half of the residential care facilities in the United States have a plan for an influenza pandemic [4].

Those plans are a solid foundation to expand the preparedness for other infectious outbreaks. Preparations have a large psychological role when non-psychiatric facilities are concerned – families and relatives of those housed at such facilities (e.g., elderly or disabled) will have their distress considerably relieved knowing that their loved ones are appropriately cared for in such extraordinary circumstances. Sometimes, the situation with the outbreak may suggest an evacuation of patients in residential facilities to an unaffected or least affected area and mental health providers should be able to identify and participate in decision-making process when such decisions are being considered.

Even after the crisis subsides, the outbreak leaves profound psychological effects in its wake. While little population studies exist, what is known from the population surveys in Taiwan following a SARS outbreak in 2003 suggests a more pessimistic outlook on life in about one-tenth of the population in the months following the outbreak. Pre-existing psychiatric conditions, demographic factors (age > 50), high-school education, perceived preparedness, and personal experiences with the outbreak all contributed to psychological distress [5].

Another study, from Hong Kong, on the other hand, found over 60% of the respondents caring more about the family members' feelings and about 30–40% finding their friends and their family members more supportive [6].

Those who were directly affected by the illness show significantly higher rates of psychological sequelae. Cumulative psychiatric morbidity among SARS survivors approached 60% 3 years after the outbreak, while the point prevalence at 30-months was about 33% (one in three), with one in four survivors suffering from PTSD and about 16% from depressive disorders [7]. That, in itself, is not much different from psychopathology displayed by other patients treated in the ICU for ARDS due to other (non-infectious causes) [8]. That study did not correlate psychiatric comorbidities with other consequences of the disease, such as a lingering physical disability or cognitive deficits. An Australian study of Australasian survivors of severe H1N1 influenza showed that health-related quality of life (HRQoL) was comparable to the healthy population a year after ICU discharge [9].

A study of families and caregivers of H1N1 hospitalized patients in Mexico provided some evidence of elevated perceived stress, depression, and death anxiety, particularly in caregivers who were older, or female, or in non-spousal relationships with the patient, and were in excess of levels that would have been predicted from normative population data and were generally comparable, or slightly lower, that levels reported elsewhere in ICU caregiver studies. The study, however, concluded that, contrary to widely publicized reports of "panic" surrounding A/H1N1, some of those most directly affected did not report excessive psychological responses [10].

The encouraging data that emerge in studies of both survivors and healthcare personnel suggest that most survivors and those exposed as caretakers have returned to their pre-outbreak mental health baseline at 1-year mark, provided their overall functioning has returned to baseline. For those survivors, however, who endured a severe ARDS and extended ICU stay, a majority had minor lung disabilities with diminished diffusion capacities across the blood-gas barrier, and most had a psychologic impairment and poorer health-related quality of life (HRQoL) than sex- and age-matched general population group [11].

During the H1N1 outbreak, the National Biodefense Science Board, recognizing that the mental and behavioral health responses to H1N1 were vital to preserving safety and health for the country, requested that the Disaster Mental Health Subcommittee recommend actions for public health officials to prevent and mitigate adverse behavioral health outcomes during the H1N1 pandemic. In its report, the Subcommittee made recommendations that emphasized vulnerable populations and concentrated on interventions, education and training, and communication and messaging [12]. It recognized, for the first time at a policy level, that emotional and behavioral health implications of such crisis and the importance of psychological factors in determining the behavior of members of the public argue for programmatic integration of behavioral health and science expertise in a comprehensive public health response [13].

A fairly early report following a limited 1995 Ebola outbreak in Congo identified that survivors were exposed to death and suffering of fellow patients in the hospitals and were exposed to reluctance of hospital personnel to treat them, and then often abandoned by family or friends. The survey identified fear, denial, and shame as the principal reactions among the survivors [14].

The incidence of mental health sequelae was studied in the aftermath of the Ebola outbreak in West Africa. One study found that 6% of the survivors, family members, and caretakers met the clinical cut-off for anxiety–depression 1 year after the outbreak, while 16% met levels of probable PTSD [15].

The overall mental health picture is inevitably affected not only by local cultural, political, and economic factors, but also by the presence of preceding and/or ongoing traumatic events, such as armed conflict, as a study from Sierra Leone shows. The study also indicated that behaviors associated with both Ebola risk and Ebola prevention may be mediated through two mental health variables: depression and PTSD symptoms [16].

In addition to individuals and groups in affected societies experiencing mental health consequences, healthcare workers, both domestic and visiting, are also affected by the mental health repercussions of the outbreak as they provide care to affected patients. As the visiting providers return home, they may have to deal with further psychosocial implications, including stigma and isolation [17].

The origins and mechanism of stigma are not well understood, but some research suggests that facial disfigurement of any etiology tends to be perceived as infectious, perhaps giving some validity to the theory that humans have an evolved predisposition to avoid individuals with disease signs, which is mediated by the emotion of disgust [18].

People with disfiguring infectious diseases, such as leprosy, tended to be shunned and banished from partaking in any social activities. Other highly infectious diseases with pandemic tendencies, including smallpox and plague, tend to leave disfiguring marks on the body, which make them easily identifiable as "survivors." Survivors of Ebola, in addition to lingering uveitis, can develop "white cataracts" that can dramatically change the appearance of one's eye and single them out among other individuals [19].

Some of the studies above can help us in anticipating where the most pronounced needs for mental health services may be during and after an outbreak. Before and during the outbreak, a subset of patients with disease-related anxieties and worries may require additional attention and services by mental health professionals. More importantly, during and after the outbreak, survivors, families of survivors and victims, and healthcare providers will likely be the populations most exposed to psychosocial and traumatic stress. Those will be populations added to the already existing patient load of patients with mental health illnesses. Patients who suffer from serious mental health illnesses, particularly those in residential settings, are considerably more vulnerable and will require additional attention during the process of preparation for an outbreak, including evacuation, if appropriate.

At the community level, psychosocial needs during the preparation phase will focus on managing the emotional contagion, addressing the concerns of the public while providing accurate information and reducing the gap between public attitudes and epidemiological facts. Preparation for public interventions in the aftermath may include the program to address the stigma that may arise surrounding survivors and their families, as well as the families of those who succumbed to the illness.

In preparing for a pandemic outbreak of an infectious illness, mental health experts and providers can be instrumental at several levels:

- Ensure that existing mental health patients are prepared and provided with both useful information and emergency supplies in case of infrastructure disruptions.
- Work with public health officials on formulating culturally competent, appropriate public communications with adequate information sufficient to mobilize and motivate for preparation, but reassuring enough to mitigate panic and despair (this includes immunization efforts).

- Work with public health officials and health facilities to provide adequate mental health support for patients in isolation and individuals in quarantine.
- Identify and suggest temporary evacuation (in case of residential care) as a possible effective, short-term solution to mitigate the effects of an outbreak.
- Work with healthcare facilities and local health officials to ensure adequate psychosocial and other support for healthcare personnel [20].
- Anticipate, to the extent possible, the mental health needs of the community during the aftermath, with an understanding that resources should likely be focused on the following:
  - Survivors of the infection
  - Families and non-professional caretakers of both survivors and the deceased
  - Healthcare providers, particularly ones caring for the critically ill
- Identify and train frontline providers to recognize signs of traumatic stress and to provide psychological first aid while providing medical care to the affected individuals and communities.
- Understand, if applicable, how significant trauma that either precedes or follows an outbreak (e.g., armed conflict, terrorism, and natural disasters) can further complicate the structure of psychological needs during and after an infectious disease outbreak.
- Understand and plan to fully utilize communication infrastructure, if available, by fostering online communication and by utilizing social media in the process of preparation before, and mitigation of the impact during and after the outbreak.
- Understand and plan for a possible failure of communication infrastructure and how to address the information deficits in that context.

At the same time, it is essential to keep an eye at what awaits the community at the other side of an outbreak, once it subsides. To that end, mental health professionals can outline plans for the following:

- Prepare for a rapid reestablishment of mental health services for pre-existing patients.
- Identify potential immediate and long-term neuropsychiatric sequelae of the infection among survivors and prepare a plan to address those issues and mitigate possible psychiatric disability as well as the public stigma surrounding the survivors.
- Identify and prepare to address the psychosocial needs of families of survivors who may be dealing with prolonged stress, exhaustion, survivors' disability, and public stigma.
- Identify and prepare to address the psychosocial needs of families of victims who may be dealing with grief, existential loss of support or sustenance, posttraumatic stress, and public stigma.
- Identify psychosocial stress in the aftermath of an outbreak in previously healthy individuals and prepare supportive measures.
- Prepare follow-up and support for healthcare providers who may fail to initially appreciate the severity of psychological trauma they have been exposed to during the outbreak.

References

1. Page LA, Seetharaman S, Suhail I, Wessely S, Pereira J, Rubin GJ. Using electronic patient records to assess the impact of swine flu (influenza H1N1) on mental health patients. J Ment Health. 2011;20(1):60–9. https://doi.org/10.3109/09638237.2010.542787.
2. Brannen DE, Branum M, Pawani S, Miller S, Bowman J, Clare T. Medical allocations to persons with special needs during a bioterrorism event. Online J Public Health Inform. 2016;8(3):e200. https://doi.org/10.5210/ojphi.v8i3.6977.
3. Hughes FA. H1N1 pandemic planning in a mental health residential facility. J Psychosoc Nurs Ment Health Serv. 2010;48(3):37–41. https://doi.org/10.3928/02793695-20100202-02.

4. Lum HD, Mody L, Levy CR, Ginde AA. Pandemic influenza plans in residential care facilities. J Am Geriatr Soc. 2014;62(7):1310–6. https://doi.org/10.1111/jgs.12879. Epub 2014 May 22. PubMed PMID: 24852422; PubMed Central PMCID: PMC4107066.

5. Peng EY-C, Lee M-B, Tsai S-T, Yang C-C, Morisky DE, Tsai L-T, Weng YL, Lyu S-Y. Population-based post-crisis psychological distress: an example from the SARS outbreak in Taiwan. J Formos Med Assoc. 2010;109(7):524–32. https://doi.org/10.1016/S0929-6646(10)60087-3.

6. Lau JT, Yang X, Tsui HY, Pang E, Wing YK. Positive mental health-related impacts of the SARS epidemic on the general public in Hong Kong and their associations with other negative impacts. J Infect. 2006;53(2):114–24. Epub 2005 Dec 15.

7. Mak IW, Chu CM, Pan PC, Yiu MG, Chan VL. Long-term psychiatric morbidities among SARS survivors. Gen Hosp Psychiatry. 2009;31(4):318–26. https://doi.org/10.1016/j.genhosppsych.2009.03.001. Epub 2009 Apr 15.

8. Davydow DS, Desai SV, Needham DM, Bienvenu OJ. Psychiatric morbidity in survivors of the acute respiratory distress syndrome: a systematic review. Psychosom Med. 2008;70(4):512–9. https://doi.org/10.1097/PSY.0b013e31816aa0dd. Epub 2008 Apr 23. Review.

9. Skinner EH, Haines KJ, Howe B, Hodgson CL, Denehy L, McArthur CJ, Seller D, Di Marco E, Mulvany K, Ryan DT, Berney S. Health-related quality of life in Australasian survivors of H1N1 influenza undergoing mechanical ventilation. A multicenter cohort study. Ann Am Thorac Soc. 2015;12(6):895–903. https://doi.org/10.1513/AnnalsATS.201412-568OC.

10. Elizarrarás-Rivas J, Vargas-Mendoza JE, Mayoral-García M, Matadamas-Zarate C, Elizarrarás-Cruz A, Taylor M, Agho K. Psychological response of family members of patients hospitalised for influenza A/H1N1 in Oaxaca, Mexico. BMC Psychiatry. 2010;10(104). https://doi.org/10.1186/1471-244X-10-104.

11. Luyt CE, Combes A, Becquemin MH, Beigelman-Aubry C, Hatem S, Brun AL, Zraik N, Carrat F, Grenier PA, Richard JM, Mercat A, Brochard L, Brun-Buisson C, Chastre J, REVA Study Group. Long-term outcomes of pandemic 2009 influenza A(H1N1)-associated severe ARDS. Chest. 2012;142(3):583–92. https://doi.org/10.1378/chest.11-2196.

12. Integration of mental and behavioral health in federal disaster preparedness, response, and recovery: assessment and recom-

mendations, a report of the disaster mental health subcommittee of the National Biodefense Science Board, adopted by the National Biodefense Science Board. 2010 Sept 22. https://www.phe.gov/Preparedness/legal/boards/nprsb/meetings/Documents/dmhreport1010.pdf

13. Pfefferbaum B, Flynn B, Schonfeld D, Brown L, Jacobs GA, Dodgen D, Donato D, Kaul R, Stone B, Norwood AE, Reissman D, Herrmann J, Hobfoll S, Jones R, Ruzek J, Ursano R, Taylor RJ, Lindley D. The integration of mental and behavioral health into disaster preparedness, response, and recovery. Disaster Med Public Health Prep. 2012;6:60–6. https://doi.org/10.1001/dmp.2012.1.

14. De Roo A, Ado B, Rose B, Guimard Y, Fonck K, Colebunders R. Survey among survivors of the 1995 Ebola epidemic in Kikwit, Democratic Republic of Congo: their feelings and experiences. Tropical Med Int Health. 1998;3(11):883–5.

15. Jalloh MF, Li W, Bunnell RE, Ethier KA, O'Leary A, Hageman KM, Sengeh P, Jalloh MB, Morgan O, Hersey S, Marston BJ, Dafae F, Redd JT. Impact of Ebola experiences and risk perceptions on mental health in Sierra Leone, July 2015. BMJ Glob Health. 2018;3(2):e000471. https://doi.org/10.1136/bmjgh-2017-000471. eCollection 2018. PubMed PMID: 29607096; PubMed Central PMCID: PMC5873549.

16. Betancourt TS, Brennan RT, Vinck P, VanderWeele TJ, Spencer-Walters D, Jeong J, Akinsulure-Smith AM, Pham P. Associations between mental health and Ebola-related health behaviors: a regionally representative cross-sectional survey in post-conflict Sierra Leone. PLoS Med. 2016;13(8):e1002073. https://doi.org/10.1371/journal.pmed.1002073. eCollection 2016 Aug. PubMed PMID: 27505186; PubMed Central PMCID: PMC4978463.

17. Chiappelli F, Bakhordarian A, Thames AD, Du AM, Jan AL, Nahcivan M, Nguyen MT, Sama N, Manfrini E, Piva F, Rocha RM, Maida CA. Ebola: translational science considerations. J Transl Med. 2015;13:11. https://doi.org/10.1186/s12967-014-0362-3. Review. PubMed PMID: 25592846; PubMed Central PMCID: PMC4320629.

18. Ryan S, Oaten M, Stevenson RJ, Case TI. Facial disfigurement is treated like an infectious disease. Evol Hum Behav. 2012;33(6):639–46, ISSN 1090-5138. https://doi.org/10.1016/j.evolhumbehav.2012.04.001.

19. Steptoe PJ, Scott JT, Baxter JM, Parkes CK, Dwivedi R, Czanner G, Vandy MJ, Momorie F, Fornah AD, Komba P, Richards J, Sahr F, Beare NAV, Semple MG. Novel retinal lesion in Ebola survivors, Sierra Leone, 2016. Emerg Infect Dis. 2017;23(7):1102–9. https://doi.org/10.3201/eid2307.161608.
20. Manderscheid RW. Preparing for pandemic avian influenza: ensuring mental health services and mitigating panic. Arch Psychiatr Nurs. 2007;21(1):64–7.

Chapter 7
Neuropsychiatric Complications of Infectious Outbreaks

Damir Huremović

Neuropsychiatric complications of infectious outbreaks have, so far, been benign in terms of proportion and scale. Those illnesses that are present on a global scale and meet the criteria for pandemics have had a very small proportion of direct neuropsychiatric involvement and subsequent complications. Those illnesses that affect the CNS in a significant proportion of cases have had outbreaks on a limited scale. A problem could arise should a rapidly spreading pandemic with a high percentage of direct neuropsychiatric complications appear on the horizon.

HIV does tend to have a significant effect on the brain, both in terms of cognitive impairment (dementia) and in terms of psychiatric complications (mood disorder). This likely stems from the direct impact on the brain tissue as well as from environmental stressors and chronic illness [1].

The problem that develops from this CNS involvement that we can learn from our experiences with HIV, is that affected patients, in addition to other impairments, tend to

D. Huremović (✉)
North Shore University Hospital, Manhasset, NY, USA
e-mail: dhuremov@northwell.edu

© Springer Nature Switzerland AG 2019   77
D. Huremović (ed.), *Psychiatry of Pandemics*,
https://doi.org/10.1007/978-3-030-15346-5_7

provide quite poor self-care and are dependent on external resources to often adhere to basic treatment [2].

A predilection for the development of mental illness can also be associated with the treatment of infectious outbreaks. A nested case-control study from the UK demonstrated that recurrent antibiotic exposure, particularly penicillines and quinolones, has been associated with an increased risk for depression and anxiety (odds ratio 1.56) [3].

Treatment with some antiretroviral agents can also lead to neuropsychiatric complications. Risks of such side effects may sometimes be offset by the seriousness of the illness they treat, as is the case of efavirenz and treatment of HIV. In some other cases, however, the use of agents such as oseltamivir, recommended by WHO and utilized for the prevention of flu outbreaks (2005, 2009), has resulted in a significant number of neuropsychiatric complications, and it remains one example where risks minimize and neutralize the benefits of treatment and lead to discord in public sentiment and general mistrust toward public health policies in an outbreak [4].

Ebola post-viral syndrome is a set of symptoms characterized by joint and muscle pain, eye problems, including blindness, various neurological problems, and other symptoms that can render the survivor disabled for a prolonged period of time [5].

A study of Ebola survivors from Guinea in form of a questionnaire found a substantial number of convalescents experiencing difficulty with concentration (37.5%) or memory (21.3%) during the subacute recovery period (defined as 91–210 days) [6]. A larger, longitudinal study from Liberia on a cohort of 150 survivors identified weakness, headache, memory loss, depressed mood, and myalgia as the most common persisting symptoms [7]. Common neurological findings in this population were impairments of either pursuits or saccades (nearly two-thirds of the cohort); tremor, abnormal reflexes, or abnormal sensory findings in a third; and frontal release signs in a sixth. Less frequently, survivors were exhibiting focal deficits consistent with stroke or parkinsonian syndrome with rigidity. Based on these findings, there appears to be a subset of survivors who have more severe neurologic manifestations that persist after acute EVD infection [7]. Neurological deficits can persist for several years after surviving Ebola, rendering survivors dependent on care and support provided by others. In addition to fatigue and those various sensorimotor deficits, survivors can experience depression (OR – 4.11) and anxiety (OR 2.33) [8].

Nipah is a virus endemic to Southeast Asia that has caused several small outbreaks in Malaysia, Bangladesh, and other countries [9]. With varied transmission modes and high case fatality rate, it is currently on the list of Disease X candidates. Nipah infection tends to cause acute encephalitis, characterized by drowsiness, disorientation, signs of brainstem dysfunction, convulsions, coma, and death [10]. Because of limited-size outbreaks, currently there are no large-scale population-based data on long-term neuropsychiatric sequelae and disability from surviving a Nipah virus encephalitis and small studies that exist indicate persistent, pervasive fatigue among adult and behavioral symptoms among pediatric survivors [11].

Other, currently geographically limited disease agents, where a significant proportion of lingering neuropsychiatric sequelae in case of an outbreak can be expected due to CNS involvement, include the West Nile virus, enterovirus 71, and possibly Chikungunya. High CNS involvement with subsequent sequelae can also be expected in the outbreaks of diseases such as rabies, measles, and polio, which are being kept under control via global immunization programs [12].

Outside of the strictly pandemic frame, there are hypotheses that are periodically resurrected implicating infection, likely viral, in the development of serious mental illness, such as schizophrenia. Some reviews indicate that individuals born to mothers seropositive for bacterial and viral agents are at a significantly elevated risk of developing schizophrenia [13]. While the specific mechanisms of prenatal viral/bacterial infections and brain disorders are unclear, some findings suggest that the maternal inflammatory response may be associated with fetal brain injury. Maternal inflammatory activation during pregnancy, particularly the role of cytokines, remains an area of interest for researchers [14]. The epidemiology and low, but steady, prevalence of schizophrenia do not particularly lend themselves to an association with an infectious outbreak. More recently, however, there has been evidence suggesting a connection between neurodevelopmental and pervasive developmental disorders (such as autism spectrum disorder) and maternal immune activation [15]. Given a recent increase in the recognition and diagnosis of autism spectrum disorders, speculation of a link between an inapparent, subclinical outbreak of a mild infectious disease and autism spectrum disorder certainly makes more sense than speculations about the link between the immunization and the autism.

Other studies, such as the Danish population-based cohort study with linkage, found that individuals who have had a hospital contact with infection are more likely to develop schizophrenia (relative risk [RR] = 1.41; 95% CI: 1.32–1.51) than individuals who had not had such a hospital contact. Bacterial infection was the type of infection that was associated with the highest risk of schizophrenia (RR = 1.63; 95% CI: 1.47–1.82) [16]. A more robust, population-based study from the same country, encompassing over a million individuals born between 1995 and 2012, found that serious infections requiring hospitalizations were associated with subsequent increased risk of having a diagnosis of a mental disorder (HRR of 1.84 (95% CI, 1.69–1.99) [17]. Even having less serious infections, but requiring treatment with antibiotics, was associated with increased risk of having a diagnosis of a mental disorder (HRR, 1.40; 95% CI, 1.29–1.51). In this study, the range of identified psychiatric disorders was fairly broad, encompassing schizophrenia spectrum disorders, obsessive-compulsive disorder, personality and behavior disorders, mental retardation, autistic spectrum disorder, attention-deficit/hyperactivity disorder, oppositional defiant disorder and conduct disorder, and tic disorders [18].

The outbreak of Zika has had a limited and specific effects on mental health, mostly on mothers or parents of affected infants and in the realm of general awareness, factual knowledge, and attitudes [15]. A small research from Brazil found that microcephaly is a factor significantly associated with high levels of anxiety and low scores in the psychological domain during the first 24 hours after birth [19].

This is an example of the indirect effects of neurodevelopmental consequences on families, caretakers, and parents. A need to provide services and support now expands to include not only patients but mothers of affected infants and expectant mothers. This need still remains significant, particularly since some of the vulnerable populations are at risk because of limited support: single mothers, with lower socioeconomic status, with lower education, and from rural areas [20].

While there are long-term studies or available evidence regarding mental health issues of parents (mothers) of infants born with Zika-induced microcephaly, there is research concerning awareness, public communication, and the use of social media which transcends direct neuropsychiatric involvement and shifts our attention towards emotional epidemiology. One study found that, for example, 30% of pregnant women who traveled from New York to Zika-affected areas were unaware of Zika-related travel advisories [21].

Although social media may come to mind as a very convenient vehicle for health information pertaining to an outbreak, a study examining Instagram posts on Zika found that 60% of the posts included misleading, incomplete, or unclear information about the virus and that over 50% of the images used expressed fear and negative sentiment, which in the long run may have affected public attitudes [22].

A Zika surveillance program in NYC was established to address the issue of Zika, as New York City sees a lot of travel to and from affected areas. DOHMH's response has focused on:

1. Educating the public and medical providers about Zika virus risks, transmission, and prevention strategies, particularly in areas with large populations of immigrants from areas with ongoing Zika virus transmission
2. Identifying and diagnosing suspected cases; monitoring pregnant women with Zika virus infection and their fetuses and infants

In its initial 6 months in 2016, it tested over 3600 patients, 5% of whom tested positive, and 11% among them being pregnant (20 cases) [23].

This possibly indicates that even serious neuropsychiatric complications in offspring may not always be motivating and mobilizing individuals and cohorts to more carefully and consciously consider such risks. Both public health planners, care providers, and at-risk individuals and communities, may not be aware of neuropsychiatric complications of an illness during the early stages of the outbreak. Unlike in the zombie apocalypse scenario, affected communities may tend to underestimate the seriousness of neuropsychiatric issues until well after the fact – during the aftermath, when lingering cognitive or neurological complications among survivors may become apparent, leading to the second wave of trauma and grief, and possibly stigma, isolation, and persecution.

Translating scientific knowledge into practical public health measures in a timely fashion and adequately preparing to prevent and mitigate neuropsychiatric sequelae of a fomenting outbreak can represent a crucial step in reducing the long-term consequences and long-term costs of such an event.

References

1. Krebs FC, Ross H, McAllister J, Wigdahl B. HIV-1-associated central nervous system dysfunction. Adv Pharmacol. 2000;49:315–85. Review
2. Eller LS, Corless I, Bunch EH, Kemppainen J, Holzemer W, Nokes K, Portillo C, Nicholas P. Self-care strategies for depressive symptoms in people with HIV disease. J Adv Nurs. 2005;51(2):119–30.
3. Lurie I, Yang YX, Haynes K, Mamtani R, Boursi B. Antibiotic exposure and the risk for depression, anxiety, or psychosis: a nested case-control study. J Clin Psychiatry. 2015;76(11):1522–8. https://doi.org/10.4088/JCP.15m09961.
4. Gupta YK, Meenu M, Mohan P. The Tamiflu fiasco and lessons learnt. Indian J Pharm. 2015;47(1):11–6. https://doi.org/10.4103/0253-7613.150308. PubMed PMID: 25821304; PubMed Central PMCID: PMC4375804.

5. Scott JT, Sesay FR, Massaquoi TA, Idriss BR, Sahr F, Semple MG. Post-Ebola syndrome, Sierra Leone. Emerg Infect Dis. 2016;22(4):641–6. https://doi.org/10.3201/eid2204.151302.
6. Qureshi AI, Chughtai M, Loua TO, Pe Kolie J, Camara HF, Ishfaq MF, N'Dour CT, Beavogui K. Study of Ebola virus disease survivors in Guinea. Clin Infect Dis. 2015;61(7):1035–42.
7. Bowen L, Smith B, Steinbach S, Billioux BJ, et al. Survivors of Ebola virus disease have persistent neurologic deficits. 2016. Available from: https://www.aan.com/PressRoom/Home/GetDigitalAsset/12003. Accessed Nov 2018.
8. Jagadesh S, Sevalie S, Fatoma R, Sesay F, Sahr F, Faragher B, Semple MG, Fletcher TE, Weigel R, Scott JT. Disability among Ebola survivors and their close contacts in Sierra Leone: a retrospective case-controlled cohort study. Clin Infect Dis. 2018;66(1, 6):131–3. https://doi.org/10.1093/cid/cix705.
9. Brown AS, Derkits EJ. Prenatal infection and schizophrenia: a review of epidemiologic and translational studies. Am J Psychiatry. 2010;167(3):261–80. https://doi.org/10.1176/appi.ajp.2009.09030361. Epub 2010 Feb 1. Review. PubMed PMID: 20123911; PubMed Central PMCID: PMC3652286.
10. Scola G, Duong A. Prenatal maternal immune activation and brain development with relevance to psychiatric disorders. Neuroscience. 2017;346:403–8. https://doi.org/10.1016/j.neuroscience.2017.01.033. Epub 2017 Jan 31. PubMed PMID: 28153689.
11. Saini S, Thakur CJ, Kumar V, et al. Computational prediction of miRNAs in Nipah virus genome reveals possible interaction with human genes involved in encephalitis. Mol Biol Res Commun. 2018;7(3):107–18.
12. Sherrini BA, Chong TT. Nipah encephalitis-an update. Med J Malaysia. 2014;69(Suppl A):103–11.
13. Sejvar JJ, Hossain J, Saha SK, Gurley ES, Banu S, Hamadani JD, Faiz MA, Siddiqui FM, Mohammad QD, Mollah AH, Uddin R, Alam R, Rahman R, Tan CT, Bellini W, Rota P, Breiman RF, Luby SP. Long-term neurological and functional outcome in Nipah virus infection. Ann Neurol. 2007;62(3):235–42. PMID: 17696217
14. Griffin DE. Emergence and re-emergence of viral diseases of the central nervous system. Prog Neurobiol. 2009;91(2):95–101.
15. Careaga M, Murai T, Bauman MD. Maternal immune activation and autism spectrum disorder: from rodents to nonhuman and human primates. Biol Psychiatry. 2017;81(5):391–401. https://doi.org/10.1016/j.biopsych.2016.10.020. Epub 2016 Oct

25. Review. PubMed PMID: 28137374; PubMed Central PMCID: PMC551350.

16. Nielsen PR, Benros ME, Mortensen PB. Hospital contacts with infection and risk of schizophrenia: a population-based cohort study with linkage of Danish national registers. Schizophr Bull. 2014;40(6):1526–32. https://doi.org/10.1093/schbul/sbt200.

17. Köhler-Forsberg O, Petersen L, Gasse C, Mortensen PB, Dalsgaard S, Yolken RH, Mors O, Benros ME. A Nationwide study in Denmark of the association between treated infections and the subsequent risk of treated mental disorders in children and adolescents. JAMA Psychiat. 2018. https://doi.org/10.1001/jamapsychiatry.2018.3428. PMID: 30516814.

18. Wiwanitkit V. Mental health of Zika virus-infected mother and mother of newborn with microcephaly. Indian J Psychol Med. 2017;39(4):546. https://doi.org/10.4103/0253-7176.211750.

19. dos Santos Oliveira SJG, et al. Anxiety, depression, and quality of life in mothers of newborns with microcephaly and presumed congenital Zika virus infection. Arch Womens Ment Health. 2016. https://doi.org/10.1007/s00737-016-0654-0.

20. Shapiro-Mendoza CK, Rice ME, Galang RR, et al. Pregnancy outcomes after maternal Zika virus infection during pregnancy — U.S. Territories, January 1, 2016–April 25, 2017. MMWR Morb Mortal Wkly Rep. 2017;66:615–21. https://doi.org/10.15585/mmwr.mm6623e1.

21. Whittemore K, Tate A, Illescas A, Saffa A, Collins A, Varma JK, Vora NM. Zika virus knowledge among pregnant women who were in areas with active transmission. Emerg Infect Dis. 2017;23(1):164–6. https://doi.org/10.3201/eid2301.161614.

22. Seltzer EK, Horst-Martz E, Lu M, Merchant RM. Public sentiment and discourse about Zika virus on Instagram. Public Health. 2017;150:170–5. https://doi.org/10.1016/j.puhe.2017.07.015. Epub 2017 Aug 12. Review.

23. Lee CT, Vora NM, Bajwa W, Boyd L, Harper S, Kass D, Langston A, McGibbon E, Merlino M, Rakeman JL, Raphael M, Slavinski S, Tran A, Wong R, Varma JK, NYC Zika Response Team. Zika virus surveillance and preparedness – New York City, 2015-2016. MMWR Morb Mortal Wkly Rep. 2016;65(24):629–35. https://doi.org/10.15585/mmwr.mm6524e3.

Chapter 8
Social Distancing, Quarantine, and Isolation

Damir Huremović

The crucial method in breaking the chain of infection is effective separation of infected individuals and suspected or actual carriers from the unaffected populations. This break of physical contact can be achieved in several ways. When the isolation is not absolute, but rather, measures are limited to reducing and minimizing contact and exposure, the term social distancing is sometimes used. Social distancing also sometimes refers to all measures used to reduce contact, including isolation and quarantine.

Book of Leviticus, which likely dates from the seventh-century Old Testament, asserts: "As long as they have the disease they remain unclean. They must live alone; they must live outside the camp." (Leviticus 13:46: NIV)

Isolation is a method that separates ill persons who have a communicable disease from those who are healthy. Isolation restricts the movement of ill persons to help stop the spread of certain diseases. Because, in cases of serious communicable diseases, those who are ill invariably require

---

D. Huremović (✉)
North Shore University Hospital, Manhasset, NY, USA
e-mail: dhuremov@northwell.edu

© Springer Nature Switzerland AG 2019
D. Huremović (ed.), *Psychiatry of Pandemics*,
https://doi.org/10.1007/978-3-030-15346-5_8

a high level of care, isolation is most frequently implemented in healthcare facilities. For example, hospitals use isolation for patients with infectious tuberculosis. Depending on the need and the acuity, wards, units, or entire wings can be placed in isolation. If there is an outbreak within a unit or a facility, sometimes the entire unit or facility can be placed in isolation, including affected and unaffected patients, as well as the staff. Throughout history, most notably during the Black Death, dedicated hospitals were established to both care for plagued patients and keep them in isolation from the rest of the population. At the time, those hospitals were known as *lazarettos*, the first one being established in Venice in 1423 [1].

There are several forms of isolation used at healthcare facilities at present time. They range from respiratory or contact isolation to strict and high isolation that is used for highly infectious diseases. High isolation stipulates a mandatory use of: (1) gloves (or double gloves if appropriate), (2) protective eyewear (goggles or face shield), (3) a waterproof gown (or total body Tyvek suit, if appropriate), and (4) a respirator (at least FFP2 or N95 NIOSH equivalent), not simply a surgical mask. Those are the standards for highly infective diseases, such as hemorrhagic fevers (including Ebola) or smallpox [2].

Quarantine, on the other hand, separates those who are still healthy, but possibly exposed to an infective agent, from those who are healthy and have not been exposed. It is a restraint upon the activities or communication of persons or the transport of goods designed to prevent the spread of disease or pests. Quarantine has a long history, but has likely been introduced as a public health measure during the Black Death in 1377 by the City-state of Dubrovnik (then Ragusa) by making the arrivals spend a 30-day period (trentina) on a nearby island of Lokrum. This method was adopted by other maritime city-states the time (e.g., Venice, Genoa) and the period was extended to 40 days (quarantina). Why the exact period of 40 days was ultimately chosen remains unknown and the theories aimed at explaining this figure range from Pythagorean numerical tradition to Biblical references [1].

In its more modern iteration, the duration of quarantine is adjusted to a disease in question. It can, therefore, last from several hours (e.g., in case of anthrax exposure, until the individuals shed their clothes and take a shower) to several decades (as was the case with Mary Mallon, known as the *Typhoid Mary*, who was forced into quarantine for nearly 25 years).

Quarantine is a significant public policy measure that can put at odds individual rights and benefits of larger societies, cutting across public health, legal and international relations realms. Quarantine was an important subject throughout history, codified in many laws, lending its name to some of the best-known ones (e.g., The Quarantine Law from 1710 in the United Kingdom). Its global prominence was at times so prominent that quarantine was the subject of some of the first multilateral international treaties, dating as early as 1851. The International Sanitary Conferences from the late XIX and early twentieth century were formidable examples of multinational cooperation to address a global issue, resulting in treaties (such as Paris, 1912 and Paris, 1926) signed by a majority of countries in existence at the time [3].

In the United States, quarantines were introduced as a response to smallpox or yellow fever outbreaks very early during the existence of colonial towns (as early as 1647 in Massachusetts Bay or in 1662 in East Hampton, Long Island). Until the end of the eighteenth century, the quarantine legislation was the responsibility of the states; in 1799, the Congress passed the first federal quarantine legislation in Section 361 of the Public Health Service Act, deriving the basis from the Commerce Clause of the Constitution and shifting the power to protect against external threats of communicable diseases from state and local authorities to federal authorities [4].

Presently, quarantine rules and regulations are governed by section 361 of the Public Health Service Act (42 U.S. Code § 264), which authorizes the US Secretary of Health and Human Services to take measures to prevent the entry and spread of communicable diseases from foreign countries into the United States and between states. The authority for carrying out these functions on a daily basis has been delegated to the Centers for Disease Control and Prevention (CDC) [5]. CDC is authorized to detain, medically examine, and release persons arriving into the United States and traveling between states who are suspected of carrying these communicable diseases. If a quarantinable disease is suspected or identified, the CDC may issue a federal isolation or quarantine order. Large-scale isolation and quarantine at the federal level was last enforced during the influenza ("Spanish Flu") pandemic in 1918–1919. In recent history, only a few public health events have prompted federal isolation or quarantine orders. Breaking a federal quarantine order is an offense punishable by fines and imprisonment [6].

Federal isolation and quarantine are authorized by the Executive Order of the President. The President periodically revises the list by Executive Order. Federal isolation and quarantine are authorized for the following communicable diseases:

- Cholera
- Diphtheria
- Infectious tuberculosis
- Plague
- Smallpox
- Yellow fever
- Viral hemorrhagic fevers
- Severe acute respiratory syndromes
- Flu that can cause a pandemic (seasonally revised)

States and local authorities also have the power to institute and enforce isolation and quarantine [7].

In 2003, during the SARS outbreak in Singapore, some 8000 persons were subjected to mandatory home quarantine and an additional 4300 were required to self-monitor for symptoms and make daily telephone contact with health authorities as a means of controlling the epidemic [8]. In 2014, while awaiting Ebola to make arrival into the United States, CDC introduced a voluntary 21-day quarantine among the measures to guard against Ebola. Close to 200 individuals in contact with the first diagnosed case of Ebola in the United States were placed in quarantine or some form of monitoring and monitoring was introduced to providers of care returning from Ebola-affected communities [9]. In October of 2014, several states introduced a mandatory 21-day quarantine for persons suspected to be in contact with Ebola [10].

A nurse, returning from helping patients in Sierra Leone, was quarantined at Newark airport in a makeshift quarantine and legally fought her way out. She subsequently defied the self-isolation protocols and recommendations that most other individuals in a similar situation adhered to; she was well within her civil rights in doing so [11]. A different nurse also returning from Sierra Leone to Texas adhered to the isolation requirements and was hailed by the local government as "a hero." A clash between individual liberties and "greater societal benefit" is bound to play out in any future quarantine or social distancing situation, its scope greatly depending on the prevalent cultural paradigm, and, as such, requires due consideration when developing programs for mental health support in the deployment of social distancing [12].

Shelter-in-place (SIP) is a variant of quarantine in which individuals are not sequestered at a designated location, but rather are sheltered in isolation where they are located at the time (e.g., home) [13]. This approach, naturally, comes with logistical challenges, but may be more appropriate from the mental health perspective, as it tends to preserve the basic group structure and relationships among individuals and, often, their daily routines.

A simulation of a SIP effect on mental health was done in a study in 2014 found that Sheltering-in-place did not have adverse effects on mental health although supplemental analysis indicated that groups that are cohesive have an easier time. It suggested SIP as a viable disaster response strategy that does not adversely impact mental health provided group cohesion is high [14].

Cordon sanitaire (sanitary cordon) refers to the restriction of movement of people within a larger, defined geographic area, such as a community. It is created around an area experiencing an epidemic or an outbreak of infectious disease, or along the border between two nations. Once the cordon sanitaire is established, people from the affected area are no longer allowed to leave or enter it. Its use, stemming from the era of Black Death, has been more extensive in the past and cordon sanitaire is rarely used now because of improved understanding of disease transmission, treatment, and prevention [15].

In limited fashion, cordon sanitaire was used in China during the 2003 SARS outbreak and in Liberia during the 2014 Ebola outbreak [16, 17].

Cordon sanitaire may be considered a legitimate and useful intervention under conditions in which: (1) the infection is highly virulent (contagious and likely to cause illness); (2) the case fatality rate is very high; (3) treatment is nonexistent or difficult; and (4) there is no vaccine or other means of immunizing large numbers of people [18].

Challenges related to this approach are, in addition to legal and ethical ones, also of logistics nature – cordon sanitaire requires resources to effectively isolate large swaths of land and considerable populations, which may be resistant to the idea. During the 2003 SARS cordon sanitaire in China, it is possible that tens of thousands of inhabitants fled the areas announced to be encompassed within the cordon [15].

At the same time, the advantage that cordon sanitaire may have over the quarantine at a designated place is that it tends to leave the community intact, including its basic resources, commerce, and infrastructure. An intact community may have better predispositions to deal with the mental health burden of an outbreak and isolation; more so than individuals separated from their families or families separated from their communities strewn around different facilities awaiting the outcome of the ticking incubation clock.

An approach inverse to cordon sanitaire is known as protective sequestration. In protective sequestration, an unaffected community separates (sequesters) itself from the external movement until the risk for an outbreak subsides. One of the best studies of self-implemented protective sequestration is a small town of Gunnison, Colorado, which sequestered itself during the 1918 Flu pandemic. The town survived without cases recorded, although sitting on a major railway. The implementation of the sequestration, although voluntary, placed a big strain on the community's economy and illustrates the challenges of implementing social distancing measures even with the community's enthusiastic support [19, 20].

Some of the less drastic, but quite effective and more commonly used measures of social distancing today include the following:

– Canceling mass gatherings [21]
– School closures [22]
– Workplace closures [23]
– Travel restrictions

Canceling mass gatherings and, at opportune times, school closings may prove quite effective in reducing transmission rates. Travel restrictions, unless extremely strictly implemented, can delay the onset of an epidemic by 2–3 weeks [24].

During the 2003 SARS outbreak, airport screening did not demonstrate the effectiveness in preventing transmission [25].

From a psychological perspective, the consequences of social distancing are summed up in two words – isolation and uncertainty. All measures of social distancing result in various degrees of isolation. Isolation in social distancing can be quite palpable, physical (contact barriers, protective equipment, physical separation by glass or locked doors) and symbolic (separation from loved ones, inability to read facial expressions from masked faces, feel a human touch on one's skin, inability to make out a human shape underneath protective equipment). The other crucial psychological aspect of isolation is uncertainty – those who are ill in isolation are uncertain about their survival and recovery, those who are healthy in quarantine are uncertain about whether they are going to get sick, those whose loved ones are in quarantine, isolation, or unaccounted for are forced to deal with uncertainty from a different side.

To prevent the psychological toll of social distancing is to address isolation and uncertainty in the early stages of planning and throughout the implementation transmission interruption via social distancing. The selection of the social distancing method is a public health matter and should not, by any means, depend on the psychological aspects of the method used. Psychological aspects, however, should be addressed early on and budgeted for in the course of action, so that measures can be taken to reduce perceived isolation and to address uncertainties that may give rise to anxiety and despair.

Addressing the psychological aspects of social distancing likely pays dividends not only in the long term, by a lower incidence of PTSD, anxiety, depression, or substance abuse, but may pay off handsomely from the very outset, by motivating participation and enhancing adherence.

References

1. Tognotti E. Lessons from the history of quarantine, from plague to influenza A. Emerg Infect Dis. 2013;19(2):254–9. https://doi.org/10.3201/eid1902.120312.
2. Guidance on Personal Protective Equipment (PPE) to be used by healthcare workers during management of patients with confirmed Ebola or persons under investigation (PUIs) for Ebola who are clinically unstable or have bleeding, vomiting, or diarrhea in U.S. Hospitals, including procedures for donning and doffing PPE, CDC. 2015 Aug. https://www.cdc.gov/vhf/ebola/healthcare-us/ppe/guidance.html
3. Markel H. Worldly approaches to global health: 1851 to the present. Public Health. 2014;128(2):124–8. https://doi.org/10.1016/j.puhe.2013.08.004. Epub 2014 Jan 7.
4. Why did Congress pass the federal quarantine legislation? Grateful American Foundation. http://gratefulamericanfoundation.com/facts/11532/
5. Vanderhook KL. A history of federal control of communicable diseases: section 361 of the Public Health Service Act (2002 Third Year Paper).
6. Weathersbee K. Quarantine: its use and limitations. AmericanBar.org. 2008. http://www.americanbar.org/content/dam/aba/migrated/adminlaw/awardsprogram/08GSwinneressay.authcheckdam.pdf. Accessed 29 July 2018.

7. Legal authorities for isolation and quarantine, CDC page on isolation and quarantine. https://www.cdc.gov/quarantine/about-lawsregulationsquarantineisolation.html. October 2014.

8. Ooi PL, Lim S, Chew SK. Use of quarantine in the control of SARS in Singapore. Am J Infect Control. 2005;33(5):252–7.

9. Dahl BA, Kinzer MH, Raghunathan PL, et al. CDC's response to the 2014–2016 Ebola epidemic—Guinea, Liberia, and Sierra Leone. MMWR Suppl. 2016;65(Suppl-3):12–20. https://doi.org/10.15585/mmwr.su6503a3.

10. Governor's Press Office (New York State). Governor Andrew Cuomo and Governor Chris Christie announce additional screening protocols for Ebola at JFK and Newark Liberty International airports. 2014 Oct 24. Available at https://www.governor.ny.gov/news/governor-andrew-cuomo-and-governor-chris-christie-announce-additional-screening-protocols-ebola

11. Price PJ. Quarantine and liability in the context of Ebola. Public Health Rep. 2016;131(3):500–3.

12. Azad A. Innocently detained: a legal analysis of United States quarantine. 2016 Sept 1. Columbia Undergraduate Law Review Blog. http://blogs.cuit.columbia.edu/culr/2016/09/01/innocently-detained-a-legal-analysis-of-united-states-quarantine/

13. Pandemic planning: sheltering-in-place fact sheet. The Church of Jesus Christ of the Latter Day Saints. https://www.lds.org/bc/content/shared/english/safety/pandemic-planning-sheltering-in-place.pdf?lang=eng. Accessed July 2018.

14. Dailey SF, Kaplan D. Shelter-in-place and mental health: an analogue study of well-being and distress. J Emerg Manag. 2014;12(2):121–31. https://doi.org/10.5055/jem.2014.0166.

15. Quarantine and Isolation: lessons learned from Sars. A report to the centers for disease control and prevention, Institute for Bioethics, Health Policy and Law University of Louisville School of Medicine. 2003 Nov. https://biotech.law.lsu.edu/blaw/cdc/SARS_REPORT.pdf

16. Liberian Soldiers Seal Slum to Halt Ebola. NBC News. 2014 Aug 20. https://www.nbcnews.com/storyline/ebola-virus-outbreak/liberian-soldiers-seal-slum-halt-ebola-n185046

17. Rothstein MA. From SARS to Ebola: legal and ethical considerations for modern quarantine (January 9, 2015). Indiana Health Law Rev. 2015 Forthcoming;12(1); University of Louisville School of Law Legal Studies Research Paper Series No. 2015–03. https://doi.org/10.2139/ssrn.2499701.

18. Hoffmann RK, Hoffmann K. Ethical considerations in the use of Cordons sanitaires, clinical correlations. The NYU Langone Online J Med. 2015 Feb 19. http://www.clinicalcorrelations. org/?p=8357

19. 1918 influenza escape communities: Gunnison, Center for the History of Medicine, Medical School University of Michigan. http://chm.med.umich.edu/research/1918-influenza-escape-communities/gunnison/. Accessed July 2018.

20. Markel H, et al. Nonpharmaceutical influenza mitigation strategies, 1918–1920 pandemic. Emerg Infect Dis. 2006. https://wwwnc.cdc.gov/eid/article/12/12/pdfs/06-0506.pdf. Accessed July 2018.

21. Ishola, DA, Phin N. Could influenza transmission be reduced by restricting mass gatherings? Towards an evidence-based policy framework. J Epidemiol Glob Health. 2011;1(1):33–60. ISSN 2210-6006. https://doi.org/10.1016/j.jegh.2011.06.004.

22. Chowell G, Echevarría-Zuno S, Viboud C, Simonsen L, Tamerius J, Miller MA, Borja-Aburto VH. Characterizing the epidemiology of the 2009 influenza a/H1N1 pandemic in Mexico. PLoS Med. 2011;8(5):e1000436. https://doi.org/10.1371/journal.pmed.1000436.

23. Rousculp MD, et al. Attending work while sick: implication of flexible sick leave policies. J Occup Environ Med. 2010;52(10):1009–13. https://doi.org/10.1097/JOM.0b013e3181f43844. PMID: 20881626, Issn Print: 1076-2752, Publication Date: 2010/10/01.

24. Ferguson NM, et al. Strategies for mitigating an influenza pandemic. Nature. 2006;442 https://doi.org/10.1038/nature04795.

25. Cetron M, Maloney S, Koppaka R, et al. Isolation and quarantine: containment strategies for Sars 2003. In: Knobler S, Mahmoud A, Lemon S, et al., editors. Institute of Medicine (US) forum on microbial threats. Learning from SARS: preparing for the next disease outbreak: workshop summary. Washington, DC: National Academies Press (US); 2004. Available from: https://www.ncbi.nlm.nih.gov/books/NBK92450/

Chapter 9
Mental Health of Quarantine and Isolation

Damir Huremović

Patients who are placed in isolation are particularly vulnerable to neuropsychiatric complications, for a number of reasons. For such individuals, isolation is evident and physical – they are confined to limited space, their movement is limited, there are contact precautions, and everyone is rushing to complete their task at hand and get out of the isolation room. Patients in isolation tend to receive less face-to-face time because a portion of patient-allocated time is spent donning and shedding the protective gear [1].

Their isolation is deepened by the illness itself and complications arising from the infection. Those complications can include delirium, anxiety, depression, a sense of hopelessness and despair, psychological trauma (acute stress disorder or posttraumatic stress disorder [PTSD]), and cognitive impairment.

Those affected by quarantine, regardless of their health status, are likely to report distress due to fear and risk perceptions. Their distress can be amplified in the face of unclear

D. Huremović (✉)
North Shore University Hospital, Manhasset, NY, USA
e-mail: dhuremov@northwell.edu

information and communication that is common in the initial period of disease outbreaks [2].

A study of patients isolated or quarantined for MERS (Middle Eastern respiratory syndrome) found that among those who were isolated and then developed MERS, over 40 percent required psychiatric intervention, while those who did not develop the illness and were not placed in isolation required none [3]. Although small in size, this study is an example that clearly illustrates how psychological well-being and psychological needs of those placed in isolation and quarantine may differ from psychological needs of those who are not in isolation and how we should devote more resource to understanding and caring for psychological well-being of those who are placed in isolation or quarantined.

What follows is an outline of major diagnostic entities that may require special attention during isolation and quarantine.

Delirium

Delirium is a neurobehavioral syndrome caused by the transient disruption of normal neuronal activity secondary to systemic disturbances, including ones caused by an infection.

Sometimes referred to as an "acute brain failure," delirium is a state of acute, organically caused decline from a previous baseline level of mental function. It can fluctuate in severity over a short period of time and it includes attentional deficits and disorganization of behavior (hyperactive, hypoactive, or mixed). It may involve other cognitive deficits, changes in arousal, perceptual deficits, altered sleep-wake cycle, and psychotic features such as hallucinations and delusions.

Delirium has been associated with increased morbidity, mortality, cost, complications, a slower rate of recovery, and prolonged hospital stays. Longer term delirium has been associated with poor functional and cognitive recovery and decreased quality of life [4].

Prevention, management, and treatment of delirium, therefore, remain an important facet of treatment of patients in isolation due to severe infection [5].

There are various pathophysiological pathways that can lead to delirium as the end result; in cases of pandemic outbreaks, the primary culprits will be infectious agents and the systemic inflammatory responses they cause [6]. Inflammatory processes are well documented in the pathophysiology of delirium, and delirium is a considerable complication among patients in isolation [7].

It is quite likely that the first cases of delirium known to medicine as described by Hippocrates almost 500 years BCE actually referred to infectious disease delirium [8].

In HIV patients admitted to hospital ICUs, delirium affects close to 30 percent of inpatients [9], which is comparable to other ICU patients [10]. It is difficult to specify the incidence of delirium among patients isolated for various infectious diseases; it would be likely comparable to one third seen in other etiologies and perhaps significantly higher where there is a direct affinity of the pathogen for CNS.

There are a number of infectious diseases that have a distinct CNS involvement, such as HIV, CMV, HSV, meningococcus, toxoplasmosis, or cysticercosis, each with a specific pathology and manifestations. Such syndromes are unlikely to be a part of a massive outbreak and, as such, are beyond the scope of this book. Other more virulent illnesses, such as influenza and measles, do tend to cause direct encephalopathies at times, but the incidence of such cases is limited compared with overall numbers of individuals affected [11, 12].

Antimicrobial treatment itself can result in delirium, sometimes called antibiotic-associated encephalopathy (AAE). A review study from 2016 of nearly 400 cases over decades of antibiotic use proposed that AAE is divided into three clinical phenotypes:

1. Encephalopathy commonly accompanied by seizures or myoclonus arising within days after antibiotic administration (caused by cephalosporins and penicillin).
2. Encephalopathy characterized by psychosis arising within days of antibiotic administration (caused by quinolones, macrolides, and procaine penicillin).

3. Encephalopathy accompanied by cerebellar signs and MRI abnormalities emerging weeks after initiation of antibiotics (caused by metronidazole).

The first two types have a quicker onset and tend to recede with the cessation of antimicrobial therapy. The third type of delirium is slower in onset and tales longer to resolve after discontinuation of metronidazole [13].

Antiretroviral medications have also been identified as causes or contributors to delirium. Efavirenz, an antiretroviral agent used to treat HIV, has been observed to cause anxiety, depression, and delirium [14]. This property is likely based on 5-HT2A serotonin receptor agonism of efavirenz [15]. The ability of efavirenz to alter perception and cause delirium has made it a substance of abuse in some cultures [16].

Other agents used to treat infection and inflammation can also greatly contribute to delirium in patients in isolation and their ability to cause or worsen delirium should be taken into account. Such medications include anticholinergics, steroids, or interferon.

Tenets for treatment of delirium in patients quarantined and isolated for infectious etiology do not differ from approaches to delirium in general – treating the underlying cause, removing or reducing the use of agents that can cause delirium, restoration of sleep-wake cycle, early ambulation, hydration, reduction of sensory deprivation or overload, frequent reorientation, placing familiar objects/photographs in patient's surrounding [17].

Patients in isolation are particularly susceptible to sensory deprivation and isolation from social contacts that can provide reorientation, support, and reassurance. If family members and friends are unable to visit patients in isolation, then it is incumbent upon healthcare personnel to provide the much needed social contact, reorientation, and support, even at times when patients appear cognitively impaired and unable to communicate coherently. Providing contact with family members via telecommunication should be used judiciously, when having such communication is expected to have a beneficial effect on the patient and patient's loved ones on the other side. Psychoeducation about delirium, its course, treatment, and prospects for recovery can be very useful and reassuring for the family who may not entirely understand why the patient acts, reacts, or behaves in a particular way and who may be disturbed by seeing the patient in such a state and not being able to visit them.

One commonly used agent in the prevention and early treatment of delirium is melatonin. The evidence for its effectiveness is not very strong, but given that the downside of using melatonin is insignificant (or at least, unknown for the time being), it remains the most frequently used agent in doses 1–5 mg at bedtime [18, 19].

Once delirium is diagnosed and pharmacotherapy for delirium is considered, low-dose neuroleptics are usually the first-line agents. Haloperidol is the neuroleptic, a D-2 antagonist, that is most widely used, is inexpensive and easily accessible worldwide, and is available for oral, intramuscular, and intravenous administration. Other neuroleptics, both older (first generation) and newer (second generation), have been used in various settings [20].

When neuroleptics are used, they are used in low doses (e.g., haloperidol 0.5–1 mg at bedtime), which are significantly lower than the doses used for the treatment of psychosis. The risk for the extrapyramidal syndrome (EPS) is significantly lower when low doses are used. One concern regarding the use of neuroleptics is the effect they have on heart repolarization (QTc interval) and that is a parameter that needs to be monitored on EKG. Neuroleptics are not routinely used for the treatment of delirium in individuals with QTc >500 ms.

When there is direct involvement of the pathogen with the brain structures, like in the case of HIV-associated delirium, patients may become susceptible to EPS when first-generation neuroleptics are used. In such cases, the use of second-generation neuroleptics is preferred [21]. In situations where the use of neuroleptics is not possible or appropriate, such as prolonged QTc interval, or in a situation where there is an effect of the pathogen on CNS that may result in seizures, an alternative approach with valproate can be considered [22].

Benzodiazepines are not recommended for the treatment of delirium and delirium-associated agitation as they may contribute to confusion and worsen delirium [23]. Benzodiazepines are, however, considered a preferred treatment for alcohol withdrawal and delirium associated with alcohol withdrawal (delirium tremens) [24].

In the intensive care unit setting, dexmedetomidine has been proven as an agent that can reduce the incidence, severity, and duration of delirium. Its efficacy appears to extend delirium of various etiologies and includes delirium associated with withdrawal from alcohol and sedatives (benzodiazepines) [25].

Depression and Anxiety

Faced with sudden isolation and quarantine, individuals and small groups can react with fear anxiety which can give way to depression and despair or anger and acting out. Depending on the circumstances, the issue of isolation or quarantine may represent a precipitating traumatic event for the individuals involved.

Symptoms of depression and anxiety are, to a large extent, a normal reaction to a stressful situation and tend to respond to support, reassurance, and accurate and timely information about the isolation status and changes in the environment. Loss of control in such situations is a reflection of reality and may be accompanied by a more or less pronounced sense of helplessness. Empowering individuals in quarantine and isolation by including them in the decision-making process for at least certain decisions helps restore dignity and sense of self-worth in difficult situations [26].

Anxiety is an appropriate signal to a number of processes that occur within the context of quarantine and isolation. A person is faced with a sudden realization that their plans for their immediate future have suddenly and dramatically changed. They may be taken to an unfamiliar setting and separated from their social context. At the very least, they would reasonably be anxious about their own health, concerned that they could fall ill at any given time. Their anxiety will likely be worsened by the inability to conduct their affairs or to provide for their dependents. If anxiety develops in this context, it likely meets the criteria of adjustment disorder with anxiety.

Similarly, from the other side of quarantine or isolation barrier, families and loved ones of those who are in quarantine and isolation may be very concerned about their well-being, but also about their own, both in terms of health and in terms of capability to provide for themselves or dependents in the absence of the isolated person. Adjustment disorder symptoms, both with anxiety and depression, can reasonably occur among those populations as well.

When the situation of isolation and quarantine involves more dramatic events, including seeing loved ones stricken by disease and suffering, seeing patients dying from the illness, or witnessing violence and the use of force (including forceful separation), those experiences, coupled with fear for own safety and the safety of loved ones, may give rise to symptoms of traumatic stress (resulting in acute stress disorder and posttraumatic stress disorder).

SARS quarantine in Canada during the 2003 outbreak encompassed some 15,000 individuals. A survey done on a representative sample, quarantined for a median of 10 days, revealed that 29 percent had symptoms of PTSD and 31 percent had symptoms of depression. Longer duration of quarantine was associated with an increased prevalence of PTSD symptoms. Acquaintance with or direct exposure to someone with a diagnosis of SARS was also associated with PTSD and depressive symptoms [27].

Several studies examined the impact of isolation on patient mental well-being and behavior and a majority showed a negative impact, including higher scores for depression, anxiety, and anger among isolated patients. A few studies also found that healthcare workers spent less time with patients in isolation and patient satisfaction was adversely affected by isolation if patients felt that they were kept uninformed of their health care by the providers [26].

The duration of isolation is directly reflected in the severity of symptoms. Short-term isolation likely does not have a significant impact on patients' well-being, as demonstrated by a survey of patients in contact isolation in Maryland [28].

As the duration of isolation extends and as the severity of symptoms increases, the psychological toll seems to increase. Patients hospitalized with methicillin-resistant *Staphylococcus aureus* or vancomycin-resistant *Enterococcus* species infections were evaluated with the Hamilton Anxiety Rating Scale and the Hamilton Depression Rating Scale at baseline and again during hospitalization. Before the isolation, there was no significant difference between the scores of the two groups. After the isolation, however, patients in isolation had significantly higher scores on both the anxiety and depression scales at the time of follow-up [29].

Respiratory compromise during hospitalization and isolation seems to give significant rise to symptoms of posttraumatic stress [30]. Survivors of the H1N1-associated ARDS requiring ICU care in 2009 were assessed for psychological well-being after 1 year. Over half of them had symptoms of anxiety, over a quarter had symptoms of depression, and over 40 percent were at risk for posttraumatic stress disorder [31].

Basic logistics sometimes can present as an insurmountable challenge to those who are mandated into isolation or quarantine. Ensuring necessary support for persons who are asked to refrain from entering public venues can impact their willingness to comply with quarantine orders. Anticipating the simple, nonclinical needs of persons under public health surveillance includes addressing potential concerns about housing, transportation, education, employment, food, and other household issues. During the quarantine for Ebola in Texas in 2014, "contact tracers" who were commissioned to monitor temperature and check for the emergence of symptoms were also used to help the quarantined resume with their routines while in isolation, also helping reduce the sense of loneliness, isolation, and anxiety [32].

Handling anxiety during isolation and quarantine requires a multipronged approach that rests on support, reassurance, providing useful information, and solving practical issues for patients and that utilizes medications when necessary. In cases of patients with no significant preexisting issues, anxiety spells can be treated with short-term courses of benzodiazepines. While any benzodiazepines may be helpful, selection may depend on availability, half-life, and the duration of action.

Short half-life medications such as alprazolam may be helpful in panic attacks or panic-like anxiety spells, while longer-acting medications, such as diazepam or clonazepam, may be better suited for persistent anxiety. Lorazepam is a shorter-acting benzodiazepine that is available in oral and injectable forms and is metabolized in a simple fashion by direct glucuronidation, so it may represent an optimal choice for "as-needed" use. Benzodiazepines can be used for the treatment of insomnia in isolation and during quarantine, preferably for the treatment of both anxiety and insomnia.

For patients in isolation who are severely ill, the use of benzodiazepines should be critically assessed, as they may contribute to delirium. The use of benzodiazepines may be particularly problematic in patients with compromised respiratory function [33].

For patients with impaired respiratory function and those who are at risk for or exhibiting signs of delirium, the use of agents with 5-HT2A antagonistic properties may be useful [34].

Medications from different classes exhibit this property, such as trazodone and mirtazapine among antidepressants or hydroxyzine among antihistaminic drugs. These medications also have sedating properties and can be used for insomnia. Among neuroleptics, most second-generation antipsychotics also have 5-HT2A antagonism and can be used in low doses for anxiety and insomnia, even with patients with delirium or at risk for delirium.

Depression

Depression, just like anxiety, is a part of a natural response to a sudden worsening in living circumstances involving separation and uncertainty, accentuated by helplessness. Depression is manifested by depressed or sad mood, loss of pleasure or interest in otherwise pleasurable activities, and a range of symptoms that may include problems with appetite, sleep, energy, problems concentrating, worthlessness, guilt, hopelessness, and outright suicidality.

DSM traditionally requires depressed mood with accompanying symptoms to last for at least 2 weeks in order to establish a diagnosis of major depressive episode, a building block of mood disorders that would merit psychiatric attention.

In isolation and quarantine, at least in the short term, the severity of depression is unlikely to rise to this level. Depression in those circumstances would likely be a part of adjustment disorder (adjustment disorder with depressed mood or adjustment disorder with mixed anxiety and depression). Under such circumstances, depression may not require pharmacological treatment, at least not in the initial period.

Such a manifestation of depression is best addressed with supportive therapy, with reassurance, and by overcoming helplessness and isolation by way of providing accurate information and by correcting cognitive distortions and misconceptions that may accompany depressive outlook [35]. Empowering individuals to make decisions and by helping them restore or establish routines during the isolation, as well as directing them to utilize healthy defenses, including humor, may go a long way in maintaining mental health equilibrium [36].

As isolation or quarantine drag on, however, individuals become more susceptible to the development of more serious depressive symptoms. In addition to HIV, for example, one other infective illness associated with prolonged isolation – tuberculosis, also carries a significantly higher risk for depression [37].

The prevalence of depression among patients with TB is almost four times higher than the prevalence of depression in the general population [38]. Stories of TB patients with depression illustrate experiences of isolation, loneliness, and despair. When stigma becomes associated with an infectious disease, isolation tends to become far more symbolic and substantial, and such individuals are susceptible to depression [39].

When the fabric of social support is ripped by isolation, it should be patched as soon as possible with available technological means, including phones, tablets, and social media. When preexisting social support cannot be reassembled due to stigma, then it is up to healthcare providers and other volunteers to step up and fill this void.

Pharmacological treatment of depression should be weighed against the severity and duration of depression symptoms, side effects of medications, their interactions, and the length of time needed to see the antidepressant effect. Treatment with medications should be initiated when expected benefits exceed the risks and the probability of recovery without medications with supportive therapy and by removing isolation and quarantine in the near future.

In cases where depressive symptoms may be accompanied by anxiety and insomnia, the use of agents with 5-HT2A serotonin receptor antagonism may be warranted, such as mirtazapine or trazodone, even if the treatment may be aborted before the robust onset of antidepressant effects due to change in circumstances. The use of mirtazapine may particularly be appropriate for patients who, in addition to insomnia and depressive symptoms, may be having a poor appetite and with or without nausea, due to its H1 antagonism and 5-HT3 antagonism [40].

If patients are at high risk for delirium, the use of antidepressants should be weighed very critically. Traditional antidepressants such as tricyclics (TCAs) are generally avoided due to their anticholinergic properties [41].

Another option for patients with depressive symptoms, anxiety, and insomnia, but who are at high risk for delirium could be agomelatine, an antidepressant that also has properties melatonin receptor MT1/MT2 agonism. This medication is not currently available in the United States [42].

Preexisting Psychiatric Disorders

Patients who go into quarantine and isolation with preexisting psychiatric disorders should generally continue with their medications. There are no apparent reasons why patients in those circumstances alone should interrupt their care other than logistical issues. Patients on some psychotropic medications may require periodic testing (drug levels for lithium and valproate, CBC for clozapine), which likely can be done in the setting of quarantine or isolation.

Challenges may arise when patients in isolation require medication treatment or intensive care that may interact with their existing psychotropic medications. A reasonable step in this context would be to review the need for psychostimulants, medications most likely prescribed and used for the treatment of ADHD [43].

In seriously ill patients in isolation, dose adjustments may be required for a number of medications, particularly if hepatic function and renal clearance are affected [44].

A reduction of dose in renal failure is individual for each medication, but in the absence of precise references, a dose reduction by 1/3 when renal clearance of the drug is not involved and by ½ where renal clearance of the drug is involved appears prudent [45].

Lithium should not be used in cases of acute renal failure [46]. Using lithium in situations where kidneys are affected can adversely affect the situation contributing to worsening of the renal failure [47].

Depending on the circumstances, patients in such cases should be switched to other mood stabilizers or second-generation antipsychotics.

Patients on antidepressants will most likely be on SSRIs or SNRIs. SSRIs and SNRIs have generally safe pharmacological profile, but those medications can cause hyponatremia, particularly in medically compromised, elderly patients, which can further complicate the management of electrolyte imbalances [48].

Due to their platelet inhibitory actions, SSRIs have also been associated with increased incidences of postoperative bleeding. Reviews generally consider this risk to be negligible, but it may merit attention in cases of recurrent surgeries or where multiple anticoagulants are used [49].

Perhaps, most caution when psychotropic medications are concerned should be given to medication interactions with other types of medications. Psychotropic medications tend to interact with a number of medications, including antimicrobials, at several different levels.

Patients on serotonergic agents (SSRIs, SNRIs, etc.) can develop serotonin syndrome when treated with antimicrobials that have monoaminooxidase inhibiting (MAOI) properties, such as antibiotic linezolid [50] or tuberculostatic drug isoniazid (INH) [51].

At the hepatic enzyme level, there are several interactions that can happen between the antimicrobials and psychotropic drugs. Quinolone antibiotics (e.g., ciprofloxacin) can, by way of inhibiting 1A2 pathway, lead to increased levels of clozapine [52].

Other 1A2 substrates that can potentially be affected by this interaction include mirtazapine, melatonin, ramelteon, and olanzapine. Interaction in the opposite direction can be seen with rifampicin, a potent 1A2 inducer [53].

Macrolide antibiotics, such as erythromycin, are potent inhibitors of CYP3A4 and can interact adversely with neuroleptics such as clozapine and quetiapine [54]. A number of other antiretrovirals (protease inhibitors, such as ritonavir) also act as 3A4 inhibitors [55]. Some azole antifungals, such as ketoconazole, have strong 3A4 inhibiting properties as well [56].

There are volumes of references on drug interactions that should be consulted when particular and specific interactions are concerned. The above summary serves just as a general educational guidance.

Substance Use Disorders

Patients with active substance use disorders who find themselves sequestered in isolation or in the quarantine may require detoxification. Detoxification is indicated for patients with alcohol or sedatives use disorder, as well as for patients with opioid use disorders. Patients dependent on alcohol can be detoxified by using the CIWA-Ar-guided detoxification approach, mostly with benzodiazepines or less frequently with barbiturates [57]. Patients who are dependent on benzodiazepines can be detoxified by using CIWA-B measured approach [58].

When patients with opioid use disorders are concerned, they can be detoxified by using the COWS measured approach to opioid detoxification. Agents used to detoxify such patients are most frequently methadone, methadone with clonidine, or a combination of buprenorphine with naltrexone, all of which have been used in patients with HIV [59].

Buprenorphine, particularly when combined with naltrexone, may be a cumbersome combination for patients experiencing acute pain (e.g., postoperatively) and pure opioid agonists may be needed for the management of pain in such circumstances.

Withdrawal from most other classes of substances can be unpleasant, but may not require pharmacological interventions.

Approaches to substance use as outlined above may not be feasible for patients quarantined in a large geographical area or who are sheltering in place. Their access to substances cannot be reliably supervised, and substance use cannot be monitored or accounted for. Providing benzodiazepines to patients who may still be surreptitiously drinking or opioids to patients who may have independent access to opioids may have unforeseen adverse consequences.

An untried, but certainly conceivable, method of last resort would be to continue to provide patients with adequate quantities of substances they use in order to stave off withdrawal and ensure compliance with strict isolation or quarantine requirements. This approach may certainly be helpful for individuals with caffeine or nicotine use disorders. It is reasonable to assume that this approach would enhance compliance with isolation in cases of cannabis use disorders as well. There is, however, no ethical or legal precedent that would allow for such an approach [60].

Motivational interviewing (Miller and Rollnick) remains a well-known, scientifically tested method of counseling clients developed and viewed as a useful intervention strategy in the treatment of lifestyle problems and disease [61]. Motivational interviewing can be done in the context of isolation and quarantine as well, either in person or via telecom equipment.

Depending on the circumstances, it is conceivable that AA or NA meetings could also take place via telecom or internet, as it is already happening for various other logistics reasons [62].

Cognitive Disorders

Patients with cognitive disorders, including dementia or intellectual disability, require special attention in terms of care during quarantine and isolation because they (1) have limited ability to provide for themselves, (2) have limited ability to understand and comply with critically important instructions, and (3) are often congregated together in institutions and can find themselves in isolation in large groups.

This is of particular importance when we understand that individuals in residential care facilities are very susceptible to outbreaks due to the nature of their facilities. A cursory literature review will reveal dozens of reports of infectious outbreaks due to various agents, both viral and bacterial, at residential care facilities throughout the world.

The best way to avoid massive morbidity and even casualties in case of an outbreak is for such facilities to have some sort of preparedness plan in place [63].

Achieving a high degree of immunization is the next step in ensuring a relative safety of residents and staff at such facilities. This makes sense, of course, only for illnesses for which effective immunization already exists [64].

Cognitively impaired patients who reside individually may be unable to be quarantined by themselves and to follow directions, and they may depend on the care of other individuals to stay with them and care for them during the isolation period. They may require frequent and simple reminders and reorientation regarding the isolation circumstances and may benefit from repetitive instructions in verbal or visual (written) form.

Patients with cognitive deficits are often on medications that are introduced with the intent of mitigating the advancement of cognitive decline. They are also more susceptible to delirium in the context of isolation [65]. Medications most frequently used in the treatment of dementia are procholinergic drugs (acetylcholinesterase inhibitors, such as donepezil), and such drugs are not thought to be contributing to or worsening delirium. If anything, they are investigated as possible delirium treatment, but with little evidence of efficacy [66].

Another medication often used to treat advanced dementia, memantine, a glutamatergic NMDA receptor antagonist and D2 agonist, may contribute to the progression of delirium, and its continued use in isolation setting should be reevaluated [67]. There has been one reported case of delirium arising from a combination of memantine and trimethoprim/sulfamethoxazole [68].

Special Populations

Apart from patients with cognitive impairments, intellectual disabilities, or other populations placed in residential care facilities, there are other populations that require special considerations during isolation and quarantine.

Young children may not be kept in isolation or quarantine without caregivers for any extended period of time.

Adolescents may have difficulties adhering to quarantine and isolation rules and they are, with healthcare professionals, a subpopulation most likely to break quarantine [69].

Children of all ages and adolescents benefit from structured time activities and routine. Routine may be designed to resemble the pre-isolation routine or it may be an entirely new routine. If isolated or quarantined children are missing school, they should be allowed to attend classes virtually. If the school activities have been canceled due to an outbreak, the virtual classroom should be considered. Other than assigning children homework and other tasks, the use of books, media, board, or electronic games can make the isolation less daunting. The use of the internet should be allowed and tolerated, but the use of social media should be monitored for the dissemination of inaccurate, yet dramatic, attention-grabbing messages and postings.

Pregnant women are another population that requires special attention in cases of isolation or quarantine. Expectant mothers may be particularly concerned about the well-being of their babies and the effect the infection may have on the fetus. Pregnancy itself may come with some emotional lability and mood symptoms, and the introduction of infection can further complicate matters. A cross-sectional study from Uganda demonstrates that HIV-infected pregnant women show more prominent signs of depression than HIV-uninfected pregnant women [70].

The postpartum period makes mothers more susceptible to postpartum depression or postpartum exacerbation of already existing mood disorders. Performing screening and providing support and education, as one would in a regular setting, can have a significantly positive effect on mothers who deliver while in isolation.

Cultural Issues in Isolation and Quarantine

Due to the nature of modern transportation and transmission of infectious diseases, isolation and quarantine can capture individuals from minority groups in a particular area or travelers from abroad into an area that becomes quarantined. In order to reduce the sense of isolation and to promote understanding, adherence, and voluntary participation, language barrier should be overcome and cultural norms adhered to, where applicable. Members of a particular ethnic group or culture, clergy, and spiritual leaders should be recruited to help overcome the facets of isolation that can be eliminated by nonphysical contact.

References

1. Sokolova A, et al. Resident poster at Nassau University Medical Center; 2015.
2. Johal SS. Psychosocial impacts of quarantine during disease outbreaks and interventions that may help to relieve strain. N Z Med J. 2009;122(1296):47–52. Review.

3. Kim H-C, Yoo S-Y, Lee B-H, Lee SH, Shin H-S. Psychiatric findings in suspected and confirmed Middle East respiratory syndrome patients quarantined in hospital: a retrospective chart analysis. Psychiatry Investig. 2018;15(4):355–60. https://doi.org/10.30773/pi.2017.10.25.1.

4. Maldonado JR. Acute brain failure: pathophysiology, diagnosis, management, and sequelae of delirium. Crit Care Clin. 2017;33(3):461–519. https://doi.org/10.1016/j.ccc.2017.03.013. Review. PubMed PMID: 28601132.

5. Chertow DS, et al. Ebola virus disease in West Africa — Clinical manifestations and management. N Engl J Med. 2014;371(22, Massachusetts Medical Society):2054–7. https://doi.org/10.1056/NEJMp1413084.

6. Fong TG, Tulebaev SR, Inouye SK. Delirium in elderly adults: diagnosis, prevention and treatment. Nat Rev Neurol. 2009;5(4):210–20. https://doi.org/10.1038/nrneurol.2009.24.

7. van Gool WA, van de Beek D, Eikelenboom P. Systemic infection and delirium: when cytokines and acetylcholine collide. Lancet. 2010; https://doi.org/10.1016/S0140-6736(09)61158-2.

8. Adamis D, Treloar A, Martin FC, Macdonald AJD. A brief review of the history of delirium as a mental disorder. Hist Psychiatry. 2007;18(4):459–69. https://doi.org/10.1177/0957154X07076467.

9. Munjal S, Ferrando SJ, Freyberg Z. Neuropsychiatric aspects of infectious diseases: an update. Crit Care Clin. 2017;33(3):681–712. https://doi.org/10.1016/j.ccc.2017.03.007.

10. Van Rompaey B, Elseviers MM, Schuurmans MJ, Shortridge-Baggett LM, Truijen S, Bossaert L. Risk factors for delirium in intensive care patients: a prospective cohort study. Crit Care. 2009;13(3):R77. https://doi.org/10.1186/cc7892. Epub 2009 May 20. PubMed PMID: 19457226; PubMed Central PMCID: PMC2717440.

11. Meijer WJ, Linn FHH, Wensing AMJ, Leavis HL, van Riel D, GeurtsvanKessel CH, Wattjes MP, Murk J-L. Acute influenza virus-associated encephalitis and encephalopathy in adults: a challenging diagnosis. JMM Case Rep. 2016;3(6):e005076. https://doi.org/10.1099/jmmcr.0.005076the.

12. Crawford N, Defres S. FS043V3 measles infection and encephalitis, The Encephalitis Society leaflet. Date created: May 2006; Last updated: February 2017. https://www.encephalitis.info/measles-infection-and-encephalitis

13. Bhattacharyya S, Ryan Darby R, Raibagkar P, Nicolas Gonzalez Castro L, Berkowitz AL. Antibiotic-associated encephalopa-

thy. Neurology Mar. 2016;86(10):963–71. https://doi.org/10.1212/WNL.0000000000002455.

14. Asselman V, Thienemann F, Pepper DJ, Boulle A, Wilkinson RJ, Meintjes G, Marais S. Central nervous system disorders after starting antiretroviral therapy in South Africa. AIDS (London, England). 2010;24(18). https://doi.org/10.1097/QAD.0b013e328340fe76.

15. Gatch MB, Kozlenkov A, Huang R-Q, Yang W, Nguyen JD, González-Maeso J, Rice KC, France CP, Dillon GH, Forster MJ, Schetz JA. The HIV antiretroviral drug efavirenz has LSD-like properties. Neuropsychopharmacology. 2013;38(12):2373–84. https://doi.org/10.1038/npp.2013.135.

16. 'No Turning Back': teens abuse HIV drugs, By JIM SCIUTTO, DURBAN, South Africa, April 6, 2009. ABC News. https://abcnews.go.com/Health/MindMoodNews/story?id=7227982&page=1. Accessed July 2018.

17. Teale EA, Siddiqi N, Clegg A, Todd OM, Young J. Non-pharmacological interventions for managing delirium in hospitalised patients (Protocol). Cochrane Database Syst Rev. 2017;(4):CD005995. https://doi.org/10.1002/14651858.CD005995.pub2.

18. Choy SW, Yeoh AC, Lee ZZ, Srikanth V, Moran C. Melatonin and the prevention and management of delirium: a scoping study. Front Med. 2017;4:242. https://doi.org/10.3389/fmed.2017.00242.

19. Joseph SG. Melatonin supplementation for the prevention of hospital-associated delirium. Ment Health Clin. 2017;7(4):143–6. https://doi.org/10.9740/mhc.2017.07.143.

20. Trzepacz P, Breitbart CW, Franklin J, Levenson J, Martini DR, Wang P. American Psychiatric Association: practice guideline for the treatment of patients with delirium. Am J Psychiatry. 1999;156(5 suppl):1–20.

21. Watkins CC, Treisman GJ. Cognitive impairment in patients with AIDS – prevalence and severity. HIV/AIDS (Auckland, NZ). 2015;7:35–47. https://doi.org/10.2147/HIV.S39665.

22. Gagnon DJ, Fontaine GV, Smith KE, Riker RR, Miller RR 3rd, Lerwick PA, Lucas FL, Dziodzio JT, Sihler KC, Fraser GL. Valproate for agitation in critically ill patients: A retrospective study. J Crit Care. 2017;37:119–25. https://doi.org/10.1016/j.jcrc.2016.09.006. Epub 2016 Sep 11.

23. Kikuchi N, Hazama K, Imai T, Suzuki S, Yoshida Y, Hidaka S. Assessment of the relationship between hypnotics and delirium using the Japanese Adverse Drug Event Report (JADER)

database. Yakugaku Zasshi. 2018;138(7):985–90. https://doi.org/10.1248/yakushi.17-00221. Japanese.

24. Sachdeva A, Choudhary M, Chandra M. Alcohol withdrawal syndrome: benzodiazepines and beyond. J Clin Diagn Res. 2015;9(9):VE01–7. https://doi.org/10.7860/JCDR/2015/13407.6538. Epub 2015 Sep 1. Review. PubMed PMID: 26500991; PubMed Central PMCID: PMC4606320.

25. Pasin L, Landoni G, Nardelli P, Belletti A, Di Prima AL, Taddeo D, Isella F, Zangrillo A. Dexmedetomidine reduces the risk of delirium, agitation and confusion in critically Ill patients: a meta-analysis of randomized controlled trials. J Cardiothorac Vasc Anesth. 2014;28(6):1459–66. https://doi.org/10.1053/j.jvca.2014.03.010. Epub 2014 Jul 14.

26. Abad C, Fearday A, Safdar N. Adverse effects of isolation in hospitalized patients: a systematic review. J Hosp Infect. 2010;76(2):97–102. https://doi.org/10.1016/j.jhin.2010.04.027. Review.

27. Hawryluck L, Gold WL, Robinson S, Pogorski S, Galea S, Styra R. SARS control and psychological effects of quarantine, Toronto, Canada. Emerg Infect Dis. 2004;10(7):1206–12. https://doi.org/10.3201/eid1007.030703.

28. Day HR, Perencevich EN, Harris AD, Gruber-Baldini AL, Himelhoch SS, Brown CH, Morgan DJ. Depression, anxiety, and moods of hospitalized patients under contact precautions. Infect Control Hosp Epidemiol. 2013;34(3):251–8. https://doi.org/10.1086/669526. Epub 2013 Jan 23.

29. Catalano G, Houston SH, Catalano MC, Butera AS, Jennings SM, Hakala SM, Burrows SL, Hickey MG, Duss CV, Skelton DN, Laliotis GJ. Anxiety and depression in hospitalized patients in resistant organism isolation. South Med J. 2003;96(2):141–5. https://doi.org/10.1097/01.smj.0000050683.36014.2e.

30. Jiang YN, Zhou W, Zhao XH, Hong X, Wei J. Post-traumatic stress disorder in convalescent patients of severe acute respiratory syndrome: (1)H-MRS study. Zhonghua Yi Xue Za Zhi. 2013;93(5):366–9. Chinese.

31. Luyt CE, Combes A, Becquemin MH, Beigelman-Aubry C, Hatem S, Brun AL, Zraik N, Carrat F, Grenier PA, Richard JM, Mercat A, Brochard L, Brun-Buisson C, Chastre J, REVA Study Group. Long-term outcomes of pandemic 2009 influenza A(H1N1)-associated severe ARDS. Chest. 2012;142(3):583–92. https://doi.org/10.1378/chest.11-2196.

32. Smith CL, Hughes SM, Karwowski MP, Chevalier MS, Hall E, Joyner SN, Ritch J, Smith JC, Weil LM, Chung WM, Schrag S, Santibañez S. Addressing needs of contacts of Ebola patients during an investigation of an Ebola cluster in the United States — Dallas, Texas, 2014. MMWR Morb Mortal Wkly Rep. 2015;64(5):121–3.
33. Vozoris NT. Do benzodiazepines contribute to respiratory problems? Expert Rev Respir Med. 2014;8(6):661–3. https://doi.org/1 0.1586/17476348.2014.957186.
34. Nic Dhonnchadha BA, Hascoët M, Jolliet P, Bourin M. Evidence for a 5-HT2A receptor mode of action in the anxiolytic-like properties of DOI in mice. Behav Brain Res. 2003;147(1–2):175–84.
35. Beck AT. Thinking and depression I. idiosyncratic content and cognitive distortions. Arch Gen Psychiatry. 1963;9(4):324–33. https://doi.org/10.1001/archpsyc.1963.01720160014002.
36. Rnic K, Dozois DJA, Martin RA. Cognitive distortions, humor styles, and depression. Eur J Psychol. 2016;12(3):348–62. https://doi.org/10.5964/ejop.v12i3.1118.
37. Yilmaz A, Dedeli O. Assessment of anxiety, depression, loneliness and stigmatization in patients with tuberculosis. Acta Paulista de Enfermagem. 2016;29(5):549–57. https://doi.org/10.1590/1982-0194201600076.
38. Koyanagi A, Vancampfort D, Carvalho AF, DeVylder JE, Haro JM, Pizzol D, Veronese N, Stubbs B. Depression comorbid with tuberculosis and its impact on health status: cross-sectional analysis of community-based data from 48 low- and middle-income countries. BMC Med. 2017;15:209. https://doi.org/10.1186/s12916-017-0975-5.
39. Nita Bhalla, Isolation, depression hounds tuberculosis patients as virulently as the disease Thomson Reuters Foundation, Catholic Online (https://www.catholic.org). 2015 Mar 25. https://www.catholic.org/news/international/asia/story.php?id=59279
40. Anttila SA, Leinonen EV. A review of the pharmacological and clinical profile of mirtazapine. CNS Drug Rev. 2001;7(3):249–64. Review. PubMed PMID: 11607047.
41. Livingston RL, Zucker DK, Isenberg K, Wetzel RD. Tricyclic antidepressants and delirium. J Clin Psychiatry. 1983;44(5):173–6.
42. Fornaro M, Prestia D, Colicchio S, Perugi G. A systematic, updated review on the antidepressant agomelatine focusing on its melatonergic modulation. Curr Neuropharmacol. 2010;8(3):287–304. https://doi.org/10.2174/157015910792246227.

43. Center for Substance Abuse Treatment. Treatment for stimulant use disorders. Rockville: Substance Abuse and Mental Health Services Administration (US); 1999. (Treatment Improvement Protocol (TIP) Series, No. 33.) Chapter 5—Medical Aspects of Stimulant Use Disorders. Available from: https://www.ncbi.nlm.nih.gov/books/NBK64323/

44. Moreira JM, da Matta SM, Kummer AM e, Barbosa IG, Teixeira AL, Silva ACS e. Neuropsychiatric disorders and renal diseases: an update. Braz J Nephrol. 2014;36(3):396–400. https://doi.org/10.5935/0101-2800.20140056.

45. Wyszynski A, Wyszynski B. Manual of psychiatric care for the medically Ill. Washington, DC: American Psychiatric Press; 2005. Appendix 12: Guidelines for Adult Psychotropic Dosing in Renal Failure.

46. Lerma EV. Renal toxicity of lithium, UpToDate. 2018 June. https://www.uptodate.com/contents/renal-toxicity-of-lithium

47. Fenves AZ, Emmett M, White MG. Lithium intoxication associated with acute renal failure. South Med J. 1984;77(11):1472–4.

48. Revol R, Rault C, Polard E, Bellet F, Guy C. Hyponatremia associated with SSRI/NRSI: Descriptive and comparative epidemiological study of the incidence rates of the notified cases from the data of the French National Pharmacovigilance Database and the French National Health Insurance. Encéphale. 2018;44(3):291–6. https://doi.org/10.1016/j.encep.2017.09.003. Epub 2017 Dec 14. French.

49. Sepehripour AH, Eckersley M, Jiskani A, Casula R, Athanasiou T. Selective serotonin reuptake inhibitor use and outcomes following cardiac surgery-a systematic review. J Thorac Dis. 2018;10(2):1112–20. https://doi.org/10.21037/jtd.2018.01.69. Review. PubMed PMID: 29607188; PubMed Central PMCID: PMC5864618.

50. Karkow DC, Kauer JF, Ernst EJ. Incidence of serotonin syndrome with combined use of linezolid and serotonin reuptake inhibitors compared with linezolid monotherapy. J Clin Psychopharmacol. 2017;37(5):518–23. https://doi.org/10.1097/JCP.0000000000000751.

51. DiMartini A. Isoniazid, tricyclics and the "cheese reaction". Int Clin Psychopharmacol. 1995;10(3):197–8.

52. Raaska K, Neuvonen PJ. Ciprofloxacin increases serum clozapine and N-desmethylclozapine: a study in patients with schizophrenia. Eur J Clin Pharmacol. 2000;56(8):585–9.

53. Horn JR, Hansten PD. Get to know an enzyme: CYP1A2. Pharmacy Times. 2007 Nov. https://www.pharmacytimes.com/publications/issue/2007/2007-11/2007-11-8279. Accessed July 2018.

54. Cohen LG, Chesley S, Eugenio L, Flood JG, Fisch J, Goff DC. Erythromycin-induced clozapine toxic reaction. Arch Intern Med. 1996;156(6):675–7.

55. Herrington JD. Common medications classified as weak, moderate and strong inhibitors of CYP3A4. Evidence-Based Medicine Consult. 2015 Oct. https://www.ebmconsult.com/articles/medications-inhibitors-cyp3a4-enzyme

56. Spina E, De Leon J. Metabolic drug interactions with newer antipsychotics: a comparative review. Basic Clin Pharmacol Toxicol. 2007;100:4–22. https://doi.org/10.1111/j.1742-7843.2007.00017.x.

57. Manasco A, Chang S, Larriviere J, Hamm LL, Glass M. Alcohol withdrawal. South Med J. 2012;105(11):607–12. https://doi.org/10.1097/SMJ.0b013e31826efb2d. Review.

58. Busto UE, Sykora K, Sellers EM. A clinical scale to assess benzodiazepine withdrawal. J Clin Psychopharmacol. 1989;9(6):412–6.

59. Umbricht A, Hoover DR, Tucker MJ, Leslie JM, Chaisson RE, Preston KL. Opioid detoxification with buprenorphine, clonidine, or methadone in hospitalized heroin-dependent patients with HIV infection. Drug Alcohol Depend. 2003;69(3):263–72.

60. Walker T. Giving addicts their drug of choice: the problem of consent. Bioethics. 2008;22(6):314–20. https://doi.org/10.1111/j.1467-8519.2008.00647.x.

61. Rubak S, Sandbæk A, Lauritzen T, Christensen B. Motivational interviewing: a systematic review and meta-analysis. Br J Gen Pract. 2005;55(513):305–12.

62. Virtual AA meetings—A new frontier or an international Clubhouse? Alcoholics anonymous, Central European Region. 2013 Sept. https://alcoholics-anonymous.eu/virtual-aa-meetings-a-new-frontier-or-an-international-clubhouse/. Accessed July 2018.

63. Lum HD, Mody L, Levy CR, Ginde AA. Pandemic influenza plans in residential care facilities. J Am Geriatr Soc. 2014;62(7):1310–6. https://doi.org/10.1111/jgs.12879. Epub 2014 May 22. PubMed PMID: 24852422; PubMed Central PMCID: PMC4107066.

64. Vyas A, Ingleton A, Huhtinen E, Hope K, Najjar Z, Gupta L. Influenza outbreak preparedness: lessons from outbreaks in residential care facilities in 2014. Commun Dis Intell Q Rep. 2015;39(2):E204–7.

65. Fick DM, Agostini JV, Inouye SK. Delirium superimposed on dementia: a systematic review. J Am Geriatr Soc. 2002;50:1723–32. https://doi.org/10.1046/j.1532-5415.2002.50468.x.
66. Liptzin B, Laki A, Garb JL, Fingeroth R, Krushell R. Donepezil in the prevention and treatment of post-surgical delirium. Am J Geriatr Psychiatry. 2005;13(12):1100–6, ISSN 1064-7481. https://doi.org/10.1097/00019442-200512000-00010.
67. Witter D, McCord M, Suryadevara U. Delirium associated with memantine use in a patient with vascular dementia. J Clin Psychopharmacol. 2015;35(6):736–7. https://doi.org/10.1097/JCP.0000000000000420.
68. Moellentin D, Picone C, Leadbetter E. Memantine-induced myoclonus and delirium exacerbated by trimethoprim. Ann Pharmacother. 2008;42(3):443–7. https://doi.org/10.1345/aph.1K619.
69. DiGiovanni C, Conley J, Chiu D, Zaborski J. Factors influencing compliance with quarantine in Toronto during the 2003 SARS outbreak. Biosecur Bioterror. 2004;2(4):265–72.
70. Natamba BK, Achan J, Arbach A, Oyok TO, Ghosh S, Mehta S, Stoltzfus RJ, Griffiths JK, Young SL. Reliability and validity of the center for epidemiologic studies-depression scale in screening for depression among HIV-infected and -uninfected pregnant women attending antenatal services in northern Uganda: a cross-sectional study. BMC Psychiatry. 2014;14:303. https://doi.org/10.1186/s12888-014-0303-y. PubMed PMID: 25416286; PubMed Central PMCID: PMC4260190.

Chapter 10
Quarantine and Isolation: Effects on Healthcare Workers

Damir Huremović

Healthcare workers bear a particular psychological and emotional brunt in the context of isolations and quarantine, including both being quarantined and caring for patients in isolation, sometimes both – quarantined on isolation wards and caring for critically ill patients in isolation. Sometimes they find in such situations voluntarily, and sometimes it happens by circumstances – quarantine and isolation orders go into effect while they are at work, and they find themselves quarantined and mandated to continue providing care while cut off from their loved ones and their everyday lives. They are in a situation to help and care for others while being exposed to the illness itself.

The burden of an outbreak on healthcare providers is yet to receive its due attention. During and in the aftermath of an outbreak, about one in six healthcare providers to affected patients develop significant stress symptoms [1]. Fortunately, even without significant interventions, those symptoms tend to remit over time and give place to everyday life and work stressors [2].

D. Huremović (✉)
North Shore University Hospital, Manhasset, NY, USA
e-mail: dhuremov@northwell.edu

© Springer Nature Switzerland AG 2019
D. Huremović (ed.), *Psychiatry of Pandemics*,
https://doi.org/10.1007/978-3-030-15346-5_10

Another study found about 11% caretakers have developed stress–reaction symptoms, such as anxiety, depression, hostility, and somatization. Particularly affected was a population of providers who were mandated to work, sometimes for extended periods of time, on specialized units due to provider shortage [3].

Healthcare workers in such situations are subject to additional stress due to their involvement in the event. They may be concerned about their health and the health of their families. They may fear contagion, be concerned about the safety of coworkers and peers in the healthcare field, and face loneliness and demanding expectations which could result in anger, anxiety, and stress related to the uncertainty of the event.

In the case of SARS, about 10% of the healthcare providers had experienced high levels of posttraumatic stress symptoms since the outbreak in 2003. Those who had been quarantined, however, those who worked on SARS wards, or had friends or close relatives who contracted SARS, were two to three times more likely to have high posttraumatic symptom levels compared with those without these exposures [4].

Even 3 years after the SARS outbreak, the experience of being quarantined or having worked in high-risk locations such as SARS wards during the outbreak resulted in higher alcohol use symptom counts among healthcare workers [5].

In yet another study from Taiwan during the SARS outbreak, the occurrence of psychiatric symptoms was linked to direct exposure to SARS patient care, previous mood disorder history, younger age, and perceived negative feelings. The most prevalent symptoms in those providers were depression and insomnia. Significant reduction in mood ratings, insomnia rate, and perceived negative feelings, as well as increasing knowledge and understanding of SARS, developing among participants toward the end of the study (and the outbreak) indicated a possibility that a psychological adaptation had occurred [6].

Despite limited resources and opportunities, there are several studies that attempted to understand some of the factors that may act detrimentally to psychological adaptation as well as those that foster psychological adaptation to working on isolation units or in quarantine.

A post-SARS study of healthcare workers in Toronto identified the following factors as likely to cause psychological distress among healthcare workers caring for patients in isolation:

(a) Perception of risk to themselves
(b) Impact of the SARS crisis on their work life
(c) Depressive affect
(d) Working in a high-risk unit
(e) Caring for only one SARS patient vs. caring for multiple SARS patients [7]

The last finding is somewhat surprising, and it may indicate either mastery through repeated experience or disengagement through repeated exposure.

Another survey from Toronto after SARS found that more contact with patients with higher severity illness resulted in higher Impact of Event Scale scores (a measurement of traumatic distress). As nurses tended to have most contact with such patients, their exposure and scores tended to be higher compared with other healthcare workers. Three factors were identified as having an effect on the Impact of Event Scale scores: health fear, social isolation, and job stress [8].

A different study from Singapore found about one in five providers displaying symptoms of posttraumatic stress after the SARS outbreak. Its findings were, however, that doctors were more susceptible to stress and that single providers were more adversely affected than those who were married. Four areas were found as important in this study: health and relationship with the family, relationship with friends/colleagues, work, and spirituality. Factors that helped reduce posttraumatic stress were as follows:

(a) Clear communication of directives and precautionary measures
(b) Ability to give feedback to and obtain support from management
(c) Support from supervisors and colleagues
(d) Support from the family

(e) Ability to talk to someone about their experiences
(f) Religious convictions [9]

In addition to professional coping styles, there may be some cultural differences as well. Another study from Singapore after SARS found posttraumatic stress at around 18%, with doctors scoring lower than nurses. Doctors appear more likely to use humor as a coping mechanism, while Filipino nurses employed religion and spirituality as their coping styles [10].

Surveys summarized above give us a limited glimpse into a complex psychological dynamic that happens with healthcare providers in isolation wards, tending to critically ill infected patients or being placed in quarantine. Surveys rely on voluntary responses by the subjects who may choose not to revisit a traumatic experience by participating, which leads to underreporting the incidence of traumatic sequelae in such circumstances. Alternately, individuals may perceive the isolation experience as unremarkable and disregard the surveys, leading to underreporting of posttraumatic stress among healthcare workers.

Despite their limitations and possible cultural bias, those surveys indicate that about 20% of healthcare providers have posttraumatic symptoms after working in isolation caring for critically ill patients. While some factors identified by those surveys are demographic (gender, age, and marital status) and cannot be changed, there are some other factors that transpire as a fertile ground for intervention in preparation for a future outbreak.

Clear guidelines and expectations: Factual preparedness ranks high among factors in most surveys, indicating that the existence of a clear plan, policies and procedures, and occasional drills may have a significant psychological impact as well. Knowing what is happening, knowing what the response is, knowing how they fit into the whole operation, and knowing own roles and expectations from them clearly help healthcare workers focus on critically important work and avoid anxiety-provoking uncertainty. Frequent policy changes, unclear criteria of case management, and other ambiguities during crisis create frustration, stress, and anxiety [11].

Communication: Another important factor is the fostering of communication between the frontline providers and their supervisors. It is essential that this communication be two way. Healthcare providers appreciate being provided with the ability to give feedback. It automatically heightens the sense of appreciation and support which they expect from supervisors. Open communication also reflects the concern that the supervisors demonstrate for the well-being of the providers.

Concern for the well-being of providers: In addition to eliciting feedback, it assumes focus on providers' health status, acknowledging risk for burnout, attempting to provide reasonable rest and relief, and at least generally assessing their ability to cope and what support they may need imminently.

Logistical support: This important segment includes both elements of logistics – clinical on-site and general off-site. On-site, it is important to provide healthcare workers with PPE, medications, equipment, electricity, HVAC, and other necessities for intensive clinical work. Off-site, it is critical to provide for healthcare workers' families, to confirm their safety, and to make sure that their basic needs are met. Providing communication equipment is an important element of logistical support.

Peer and spiritual support: Understanding that providers appreciate an opportunity to talk to someone, both formally and informally. They may be encouraged to talk to each other or to a designated support staff member from the outside via telecom equipment. Their spiritual needs should also be assessed and met as they spirituality can significantly foster resilience.

Psychological support: Professional psychological support may not be necessary during the isolation or quarantine work, but it should be made available to healthcare workers in isolation. They may be informed about the possibility of stress reactions and how counseling after the isolation will be made available although most providers do not need it. In some cases, however, that include preexisting medical illness and the emergence of grossly disorganized or dangerous behavior, as well as active substance abuse issues, actual psychiatric intervention may be needed.

References

1. Lu YC, Shu BC, Chang YY, Lung FW. The mental health of hospital workers dealing with severe acute respiratory syndrome. Psychother Psychosom. 2006;75(6):370–5.
2. Lung FW, Lu YC, Chang YY, Shu BC. Mental symptoms in different health professionals during the SARS attack: a follow-up study. Psychiatry Q. 2009;80(2):107–16. https://doi.org/10.1007/s11126-009-9095-5. Epub 2009 Feb 27
3. Mak IW, Chu CM, Pan PC, Yiu MG, Chan VL. Long-term psychiatric morbidities among SARS survivors. Gen Hosp Psychiatry. 2009;31(4):318–26. https://doi.org/10.1016/j.genhospsych.2009.03.001. Epub 2009 Apr 15
4. Wu P, Fang Y, Guan Z, Fan B, Kong J, Yao Z, Liu X, Fuller CJ, Susser E, Lu J, Hoven CW. The psychological impact of the SARS epidemic on hospital employees in China: exposure, risk perception, and altruistic acceptance of risk. Can J Psychiatr. 2009;54(5):302–11. PubMed PMID: 19497162; PubMed Central PMCID: PMC3780353.
5. Wu P, Liu X, Fang Y, Fan B, Fuller CJ, Guan Z, Yao Z, Kong J, Lu J, Litvak IJ. Alcohol abuse/dependence symptoms among hospital employees exposed to a SARS outbreak. Alcohol Alcohol. 2008;43(6):706–12. https://doi.org/10.1093/alcalc/agn073. Epub 2008 Sep 12. PubMed PMID: 18790829; PubMed Central PMCID: PMC2720767.
6. Su TP, Lien TC, Yang CY, Su YL, Wang JH, Tsai SL, Yin JC. Prevalence of psychiatric morbidity and psychological adaptation of the nurses in a structured SARS caring unit during outbreak: a prospective and periodic assessment study in Taiwan. J Psychiatr Res. 2007;41(1–2):119–30. Epub 2006 Feb 7
7. Styra R, Hawryluck L, Robinson S, Kasapinovic S, Fones C, Gold WL. Impact on health care workers employed in high-risk areas during the Toronto SARS outbreak. J Psychosom Res. 2008;64(2):177–83. https://doi.org/10.1016/j.jpsychores.2007.07.015.
8. Maunder RG, Lancee WJ, Rourke S, Hunter JJ, Goldbloom D, Balderson K, Petryshen P, Steinberg R, Wasylenki D, Koh D, Fones CS. Factors associated with the psychological impact of severe acute respiratory syndrome on nurses and other hospital workers in Toronto. Psychosom Med. 2004;66(6):938–42.

9. Chan AO, Huak CY. Psychological impact of the 2003 severe acute respiratory syndrome outbreak on health care workers in a medium size regional general hospital in Singapore. Occup Med (Lond). 2004;54(3):190–6.
10. Phua DH, Tang HK, Tham KY. Coping responses of emergency physicians and nurses to the 2003 severe acute respiratory syndrome outbreak. Acad Emerg Med. 2005;12(4):322–8.
11. Wong EL, Wong SY, Lee N, Cheung A, Griffiths S. Healthcare workers' duty concerns of working in the isolation ward during the novel H1N1 pandemic. J Clin Nurs. 2012;21(9–10):1466–75. https://doi.org/10.1111/j.1365-2702.2011.03783.x. Epub 2011 Jul 21

Chapter 11
Mental Health Care for Survivors and Healthcare Workers in the Aftermath of an Outbreak

Jacqueline Levin

The approach to mental health care for survivors is informed by a number of individual, social, and cultural factors. One must first consider the psychiatric sequelae of surviving the illness, its complications, and the complications of its treatments. In the acute phase of illness, even small foci of infection can produce psychiatric symptoms ranging from mood changes and irritability to cognitive dysfunction to psychosis. Neuropsychiatric manifestations may even present as the first signs of infection in an otherwise well-appearing patient. Hematogenous spread of bacteria or virus to the central nervous system can produce meningitis associated with significant morbidity and mortality, presenting symptoms including headache, nausea, nuchal rigidity, confusion, lethargy, and apathy to be confirmed by the examination of CSF. Bacterial meningitis may also result in brain abscess, with seizures and various psychiatric symptoms prevailing depending on the size and location of the abscess. Successful treatment with empirical

J. Levin (✉)
Department of Psychiatry, North Shore University Hospital, Manhasset, NY, USA

© Springer Nature Switzerland AG 2019   127
D. Huremović (ed.), *Psychiatry of Pandemics*,
https://doi.org/10.1007/978-3-030-15346-5_11

antibiotics and primary excision of the abscess may still result in persistent psychiatric symptoms. In cases of viral encephalitis, psychiatric symptoms are very common in the acute phase and recovery, especially mood disorders. Major disability can result, including symptoms of depression, amnestic disorders, hypomania, irritability, and disinhibition (sexual, aggressive, and rageful) even months after recovery. Psychosis may also rarely result. Standard treatments with antidepressants, stimulants, mood stabilizers, neuroleptics, and electroconvulsive therapy should be applied [1].

Individuals may suffer potentially permanent cognitive deficits secondary to illness or its treatments that will require cognitive rehabilitation. In cases of delirium, if the resultant encephalopathy is severe or persistent, pharmacologic interventions with antipsychotics (such as haloperidol 0.5–20 mg/day) and mood stabilizers (such as valproic acid up to 60 mg/kg/day) should be considered. In addition, psychosocial interventions will need to be implemented to maintain safety and care for someone who may no longer be able to care for themselves. Additional consideration on this topic is provided in the chapter entitled Neuropsychiatric Sequelae of Infectious Outbreaks.

In the wake of an infectious disease outbreak, the loss of functioning imparted by illness may leave survivors feeling demoralized, helpless, and in a state of mourning over the loss of the person they used to be. If the patient experiences marked distress or significant impairment in social or occupational functioning, they may meet DSM-V criteria for adjustment disorder. Therapeutic interventions in those instances should focus on helping individuals regain a sense of autonomy and mastery through rehabilitation. It is helpful to focus on gaining immediate control over some specific aspects of their lives, as well as helping the persons identify and link with agencies and supports in the community [2]. Psychotherapy, both individual and group therapy, if available, can help survivors come to terms with the loss of functioning.

If the patient is left with significant depressive symptoms meeting DSM-V criteria for major depressive disorder, the psychopharmacological approach may be warranted; selective serotonin reuptake inhibitors or serotonin–norepinephrine reuptake inhibitors should be considered in such cases. Concurrent insomnia may be treated with melatonin, trazodone, ramelteon, or any available sedatives–hypnotics. Prescribers should be aware of drug–drug interactions and cytochrome P450 interactions between selected psychotropics and medications prescribed by infectious disease physicians in treating survivors. Patients who are at increased risk of developing delirium (i.e., elderly, dementia, and brain disease) should also be monitored for changes in mental status, attention, alertness, and orientation. Psychotherapy (cognitive behavioral therapy, supportive psychotherapy, and psychodynamic psychotherapy) may also be of clinical benefit if available. Enlisting local cultural and spiritual leaders may also help build hope and confidence.

Another important consideration is that proximity to and survival from life-threatening events (in this case illness) are known risk factors for the development of trauma-based disorders, including acute stress disorder and posttraumatic stress disorder (PTSD). PTSD is characterized by intrusive thoughts, nightmares, and flashbacks of past traumatic events, avoidance of reminders of trauma, hypervigilance, and sleep disturbance leading to significant social, occupational, and interpersonal dysfunction. In the aftermath of pandemics, increased psychiatric screening and surveillance is recommended to address acute stress disorder, posttraumatic stress disorder, depressive disorders, and substance abuse.

In the short-term aftermath, psychological first aid can be administered to patients by public health and public behavioral health workers. Such interventions focus on establishing a respectful, supportive rapport, triaging critical needs, normalizing stress and grief reactions, supporting positive thoughts about the future, and teaching mindfulness-based techniques to decrease the levels of stress and hyperarousal (i.e., deep breathing, progressive muscle relaxation, and guided imagery). Normalizing angry feelings while decreasing anger-driven behaviors can also play a therapeutic role [2].

In the long-term aftermath of a pandemic, trauma-focused therapies and pharmacological treatments may be indicated. Once a diagnosis of PTSD is made, treatment should be initiated promptly. First-line treatment consists of trauma-focused cognitive behavioral therapy (CBT) to help reduce pessimistic and catastrophic thoughts about the future. Exposure therapy and eye movement desensitization and reprocessing (EMDR) therapies may also be utilized. If these therapeutic modalities are not readily available, selective serotonin reuptake inhibitors (SSRIs) and serotonin–norepinephrine reuptake inhibitors (SNRIs) can also be considered first-line treatments, to be administered for a duration of at least 6–12 months to prevent recurrence and relapse. Monotherapy or adjunctive therapy with quetiapine may also be considered. Alpha-adrenergic receptor blockers such as prazosin could be used for sleep disruption and nightmares, either alone or in conjunction with an antidepressant [3].

Special consideration should also be given to individuals with preexisting mental health issues who may experience setbacks, relapses, and impairments in functioning. More vulnerable patients with serious and persistent mental disorders such as primary psychotic illnesses or developmental disorders are likely to experience destabilizing disruptions in routine and access to medications/treatments. Psychotic, manic, or depressive symptoms may be intensified due to stress; increasing standing psychotropic medications may be indicated. Preexisting anxiety and substance use disorders are likely to worsen in the face of constant fear and distress. It is helpful to provide patients with a supply of PRN or "as-needed" extra tablets of antipsychotics or benzodiazepines as the pandemic unfolds to treat worsening symptoms. It is also prudent to enlist these patients' families and social supports to warn them of the risk for psychiatric destabilization and provide them with specific examples of worsening psychiatric symptoms to be on the lookout for. A safety plan and communication strategy should be developed with the patient and his or her family in the aftermath of a pandemic, with attention paid to potential barriers imposed by the pandemic (i.e. pharmacy closures, difficulty accessing medications). When possible, it may be prudent to prescribe a few months' additional supply of medications to be entrusted to a reliable family member. Increased monitoring is prudent in the aftermath of a pandemic with bimonthly or even weekly visits, depending on the severity of illness. For patients who are unable to access their usual providers, telepsychiatry can be a helpful substitute where available. Mental health professionals should be trained in the assessment of suicidality and safety concerns which may arise in the setting of acute anxiety, disability, bereavement, and multiple losses.

As a special consideration, it is worth noting that survivors of pandemics may find themselves the targets of pronounced stigma and rejection by their local communities. Affected individuals may blame themselves, and they may be prevented from returning to their homes or workplaces [4]. Entire cultural groups, communities, and geographic populations may become targets of stigmatization, which may serve as a barrier to seeking care [5]. In these cases, validating the experience of the stigmatized person is of utmost importance. In some communities, survivors of pandemics have been lauded as heroes by nongovernmental agencies in an attempt to decrease stigma [4]. Fostering resilience in such persons and their communities can help them to reclaim a sense of self-efficacy and fortitude in the face of adversity [6].

Just as patients experience significant emotional impacts in the course of a pandemic, so too will the brave and selfless healthcare personnel who are charged with the responsibility of providing aid to the infected. Their burden, however, is compounded by their high and persistent risk for exposure and death, separation from their loved ones which may be either enforced or due to prolonged work shifts, seeing traumatic images of their disfigured or dying patients, working during surge conditions in overburdened settings with chronically scarce supplies and medications/vaccines, experiencing hopelessness due to massive human losses in spite of their best efforts to provide care, managing human remains, experiencing workforce quarantine, witnessing the death of their colleagues, lack of reinforcements and replacements, and their own fatigue and burnout, to name a few of the many traumas they must endure in the course of their service [7].

It, therefore, does not come as a surprise that studies of nurses who treated SARS patients during the 2003 outbreak indicated high levels of stress and 11% rates of traumatic stress reactions, including depression, anxiety, hostility, and somatization symptoms [8]. One study showed that even 1 year after the SARS outbreak in 2003, healthcare worker SARS survivors still had persistently higher levels of stress and psychological distress than non–healthcare worker SARS survivors [9]. Similar findings have been reported in multiple studies indicating acute and persistently elevated stress levels as well as other emotional sequelae of healthcare workers during and after pandemic disease outbreaks [10–12]. Those findings indicate that left unaddressed, emotional needs and wounds of healthcare personnel grappling with an outbreak can reverberate long, perhaps for many years, after an outbreak has abated.

Healthcare personnel working at great personal peril will, therefore, require frequent and clear communication regarding the status of the pandemic and developments as they unfold. Communication at every level should be monitored, with systems in place to bidirectionally transmit news among healthcare workers, their administration, healthcare facilities, and the government [10].

Leadership, structure, and clear delineation of duties and responsibilities are critical. Determining staffing needs and establishing predictable schedules will lay a stable foundation for healthcare workers and ground them in the face of other destabilizing forces. Healthcare workers on the frontlines should be supported to the fullest extent possible as the pandemic unfolds to prepare for what is to come. Educational materials should be developed and provided that can outline what healthcare workers might expect in the course of their duties, including common reactions and stressors they may encounter from the public, patients, their friends and families, or from within themselves. This is of utmost importance, as an unprepared workforce may feel afraid to serve; in a survey of over 6400 healthcare workers across 47 facilities in the New York metropolitan region, only 48.4% said they would be willing to report to work during an outbreak of SARS, most frequently citing fear for personal or family safety as the reason they were unwilling to work [13].

Given the real and understandable fear of contracting illness, comprehensive and repeated training on infection control and how to use personal protective equipment can help increase the confidence of the workforce that their personal safety will be maintained. Healthcare personnel should also be offered periodic health assessments to reassure them of their physical well-being [8]. Preparations should also center on immunization programs, available vaccines for frontline healthcare personnel, availability of prophylactic medications, and assurances that their concerns and needs will be heard and met [14].

A study of the psychological impact of the 2003 SARS outbreak on healthcare workers in Singapore found that support from supervisors and colleagues was a significant negative predictor for psychiatric symptoms and PTSD, in addition to clear communication of directives and precautionary measures which also helped reduce psychiatric symptoms [15]. Buddy systems pairing more and less experienced healthcare workers can help not only to transfer skills, but also to reduce social isolation and promote a sense of support and interconnectedness [10]. The experience of being a healthcare worker during a pandemic is both isolating and stigmatizing; having a partner to share the experience with would be beneficial on multiple levels.

Administrators can improve the situation by being attentive to the psychological, physical, spiritual, and psychosocial needs of healthcare workers. Systems should be implemented for rest and relief of duties to prevent burnout; it is also prudent to limit overtime [2]. Programs promoting well-being incorporating mindfulness and relaxation techniques can help healthcare workers develop self-help skills during times of increased stress; once learned, they may also be able to pass such skills on to their patients. Workforce resilience programs and self-care strategies should be promoted. Teamwork and morale-building activities should also be promoted, as well as wellness breaks. It may also be meaningful to plan staff-appreciation events and verbally acknowledge their ongoing efforts [2]. Spiritual leaders from the faith-based community may also be called upon to provide spiritual guidance to affected healthcare workers who would find tremendous comfort in such an outlet.

It is also important to remember that healthcare workers will have their own sick family members, childcare issues, and personal affairs impressing upon them from the outside world, which can leave them feeling pulled between a sense of duty to their patients and their loved ones. Psychosocial programs that are mindful of providing services for the families of healthcare workers can go a long way in supporting staff and protecting morale. Lending cellular phones, laptops, or tablets to healthcare workers and their families to ensure they are able to maintain ongoing communication, as well as providing updates on websites and hotlines, can also help healthcare workers feel they are still interconnected with their families and may alleviate some of the real pressures that are felt. Furthermore, healthcare workers should be regularly reminded and trained in infection control measures when they return home; for example, reminding staff of handwashing and to change clothes before entering their homes to protect family members. Providing disposable scrubs or garments especially for wear in the hospital may also help decrease healthcare workers' anxiety about transmitting illness to their families back home [2]. It may also help to designate healthcare workers a specialized status within the community, given the crucial public service role they play. For example, providing specialized identification cards that might prevent them from waiting in lines at gas stations or supermarkets, as well as fair compensation and a stipend for their families, may further promote a sense of professional pride and goodwill and may help counteract the negative impact of the stigma that they may endure.

Lastly, employee assistance programs should target healthcare personnel who have developed traumatic, affective, or anxiety disorders as well as those struggling with increased substance use disorders. Increased mental health monitoring is advised, given healthcare workers' proximity and repeated exposure to traumatic experiences, as well as the well-documented evidence of the persistent distress they are likely to experience. They should be considered a high-risk group for developing psychopathology in the aftermath of a pandemic and they should be given the same consideration and nurturing of any other high-risk population identified. Healthcare workers should have ready access to psychiatric care, pharmacologic interventions, and both individual and group psychotherapy. They should be reassured that their families will receive the same.

Practitioners tasked with treating patients in the aftermath of a pandemic will face challenges in providing standard care, both due to infrastructural and crisis-related adversities, as well as secondary to unique biological changes imparted by the disease itself. It is important for practitioners to be aware of common drug interactions, dosing, and titration strategies, and special considerations for different classes of psychopharmacological agents used. This section aims to review and summarize pertinent aspects of psychopharmacological agents which may be of use to future practitioners who find themselves providing psychiatric care in the wake of a pandemic.

Antidepressants are first-line agents for a number of psychiatric conditions that may be encountered in the aftermath of a pandemic. Such diagnoses include mood disorder secondary to a general medical condition, major depressive disorder, posttraumatic stress disorder, dissociative disorder, obsessive-compulsive disorder, and generalized anxiety disorder, to name a few. To identify and treat major depressive disorder, the psychiatric interview should focus on the psychological symptoms of depression (i.e., sad mood, anhedonia, hopelessness, worthlessness, guilt, and suicidality) rather than the vegetative symptoms (i.e., sleep disturbance, appetite change, psychomotor changes, and decreased concentration and energy), which may be of lower yield in the setting of acute medical illness. Depression should also be distinguished from hypoactive delirium, which may also present with diminished appetite, sleep disturbance, and an appearance of apathy (in the case of delirium, treatment with antipsychotics will be more effective than addition of an antidepressant).

An adequate trial of an antidepressant is defined as 12 weeks of antidepressant therapy at an effective therapeutic dose. It is helpful to establish expectations with patients by reminding them that daily use is important (rather than as-needed use), that symptoms may take 2–4 weeks before they begin improving, and that common side effects such as nausea, diarrhea, headache, and sexual dysfunction may be expected. Patients age 24 and younger should be monitored for worsening suicidal ideation. For patients with significant concurrent anxiety, a slow titration may be most appropriate with temporary use of benzodiazepines until the antidepressant takes clinical effect (e.g., lorazepam 0.5–1 mg orally two to three times per day). If the drug is not working within 6–8 weeks, the patient may require a dose increase or a switch should be considered. Providers should treat until remission or a significant reduction in symptoms is observed, continuing treatment for 1 year for the first episode of major depressive disorder and indefinitely if there have been two or more episodes.

There are six principal selective serotonin reuptake inhibitors in common use: fluoxetine, sertraline, citalopram, escitalopram, paroxetine, and fluvoxamine. The global accessibility of these agents may vary. Fluoxetine has a dose range from 10 to 80 mg and has the longest half-life (2–3 days), which makes it an ideal choice for patients in whom there are concerns for compliance or consistent access to medication. Sertraline has a dose range of 25–200 mg, and its wide range of dosing making it a good choice for elderly patients or for those who may be sensitive to side effects. Fluoxetine and sertraline have no renal dose adjustment, but a lower or half dose is recommended for patients with hepatic impairment. Citalopram doses range from 10 to 40 mg, but should not exceed more than 20 mg/day for patients over age 60 or if the hepatic impairment is present. There is no dose adjustment for mild/moderate renal impairment, but caution should be used in severe impairment. It is important to note that citalopram should not be combined with other QTc prolonging agents (applies to antimicrobials such as erythromycin, clarithromycin, fluoroquinolones, antifungals, and antimalarials) for increased risk of torsades de pointes [16]. Escitalopram, an enantiomer of citalopram, has dose ranges from 5 to 20 mg, should not exceed more than 10 mg/day in the elderly or in cases of hepatic impairment, or if severe renal impairment is present. Paroxetine doses range from 20 to 40 mg, with only 10 mg/day recommended in cases of renal or hepatic impairment. It has the shortest half-life of all the SSRIs (21 hours), resulting in an uncomfortable discontinuation syndrome and may not be ideal for patients with interrupted access to care/medications. Side effects of sedation, weight gain, constipation, and dry mouth may make it a favorable option, however, for specific patients. Lastly, fluvoxamine doses range from 100 to 200 mg; however, many drug–drug interactions are associated with its use and should be monitored for.

Clinically significant interactions exist between selective serotonin reuptake inhibitors and several antiretrovirals in the setting of HIV/AIDS. For example, SSRIs shown to have decreased metabolism in the setting of ritonavir include sertraline and citalopram, but alternatively, the levels of fluoxetine and fluvoxamine are both decreased by nevirapine. Fluoxetine and fluvoxamine can both increase the levels of amprenavir, delavirdine, efavirenz, indinavir, lopinavir/ritonavir, nelfinavir, ritonavir, and saquinavir [17].

Tricyclic antidepressants have common side effects such as drowsiness, confusion, dizziness, weight gain, hypotension, and tachycardia, as well as anticholinergic side effects including dry mouth, blurred vision, decreased gastrointestinal motility, and urinary retention. Some of these side effects can be taken advantage of in the setting of HIV/AIDS, specifically weight gain, increased sleep, and decreased diarrhea [17]. Mirtazapine 7.5–45 mg at bedtime similarly may be a good choice in patients with postinfectious cachexia and exhaustion as it promotes weight gain and can cause a significant sedation, making it suitable for patients suffering from insomnia. Bupropion 75–450 mg/day can be helpful in postinfectious anergia, but prescribers should bear in mind that it lowers the seizure threshold. Tricyclic antidepressants and serotonin–norepinephrine reuptake inhibitors are useful if there is also concurrent neuropathic pain or a lingering inflammatory process that persists following some viral infections; for example, amitriptyline 10–400 mg at bedtime, duloxetine 60–120 mg/day, or venlafaxine 75–225 mg/day.

Antimicrobial drugs themselves have had prominent associations with delirium and a host of other psychiatric side effects. For example, antibacterials such as quinolones have been associated with psychosis, paranoia, mania, agitation, and Tourette-like syndrome, and procaine penicillin has been associated with delirium, psychosis, agitation, depersonalization, and hallucinations. Mefloquine and other antiparasitic/antimalarial drugs have been associated with confusion, psychosis, mania, depression, aggression, anxiety, and delirium. Antituberculous drugs such as cycloserine have been associated with agitation, depression, psychosis, and anxiety. Antivirals such as amantadine have been associated with psychosis and delirium, and interferon treatment is frequently associated with depression [1].

In addition to being cognizant of the side effects of the treatments themselves, drug–drug interactions between antimicrobials and psychotropic drugs abound. Psychiatric care providers should exercise caution when utilizing specific psychotropics (i.e., antipsychotics or tricyclic antidepressants) in the setting of other QTc interval-prolonging agents such as erythromycin or ketoconazole, due to increased risk of ventricular arrhythmias and torsades de pointes. Providers should keep in mind that linezolid is an irreversible monoamine oxidase-A inhibitor and isoniazid is a weaker monoamine oxidase inhibitor—so the serotonin syndrome or hypertensive crisis can result if serotonergic antidepressants or other sympathomimetics (such as meperidine, which is an opioid analgesic) are coadministered. Antimalarials have been shown to increase the levels of phenothiazine neuroleptics. Clarithromycin and erythromycin can increase carbamazepine, buspirone, clozapine, alprazolam, and midazolam levels. Quinolones may increase clozapine and benzodiazepine levels but reduce benzodiazepine effect via the GABA receptor. Lastly, providers should be aware that isoniazid can increase haloperidol and carbamazepine levels [1].

Psychiatric care providers should be aware of the myriad complications of corticosteroid use, seen in up to 6% of patients presenting with significant neuropsychiatric manifestations. Anxiety, mania, delirium, or psychosis may present with the administration of corticosteroids, and a dose-dependent relationship has been observed. In most cases, a reduction of corticosteroid dose will improve symptoms; however, if this strategy is not possible or ineffective, antipsychotics or mood stabilizers should be used [18]. In patients presenting with predominantly manic symptoms, special consideration should be given to medical comorbidities when selecting a mood stabilizer. Lithium may be difficult to administer in the setting of renal dysfunction, electrolyte abnormalities, or fluid shifts. Valproic acid may be relatively contraindicated in patients with significant liver disease or pancreatitis. Carbamazepine has antidiuretic actions, has quinidine-like effects on cardiac conduction, and has been associated with aplastic anemia and leukopenia which prescribers should bear in mind.

Conclusion

Providing psychiatric care to survivors and healthcare workers in the aftermath of a pandemic outbreak is a complicated, but crucial, imperative in the service of reducing the burden of human suffering. Challenges will abound on multiple levels, but there is no substitute for preparedness. Knowledge of assessment, differential diagnosis, medical complications, and treatment will aid the psychiatric care provider in developing a treatment approach for these patients who are most vulnerable during their greatest time of need.

References

1. Levenson J. Chapter 27: Infectious diseases. In: Levenson J, editor. Textbook of psychosomatic medicine. 2nd ed. Washington, DC: American Psychiatric Publishing Press; 2010. p. 615–35.
2. Havice-Cover PJ, Drennen C. Pandemic influenza: quarantine, isolation and social distancing [Internet]. Colorado: The Colorado Department of Human Services Division of Mental Health. Available from: http://www.realisticpreparedness.com/downloads/PanFluQuarantineIsolation.pdf
3. Stein MB. Pharmacotherapy for posttraumatic stress disorder in adults. Post TW, editor. UpToDate. Waltham: UpToDate Inc. http://www.uptodate.com. Accessed 16 Dec 2018.
4. Reardon S. Ebola's mental-health wounds linger in Africa. Nature. 2015;519:13–4.
5. Honermann B. An "epidemic within an outbreak:" the mental health consequences of infectious disease epidemics. 2015 Feb 26 [cited 2018 Dec 16]. In: O'Neill Institute for National & Global Health Law Blog [Internet]. Washington: O'Neill Institute. [2007] -. [about 3 screens] Available from: http://oneill.law.georgetown.edu/epidemic-within-outbreak-mental-health-consequences-infectious-disease-epidemics/
6. Missouri Department of Health and Senior Services. Pandemic influenza plan: psychosocial services preparedness [Internet]. 2018 September. [Cited 2019 Jan 11]. Available from: https://health.mo.gov/emergencies/panflu/pdf/panfluplanpsychosocial.pdf
7. Shultz JM. Mental health consequences of infectious disease outbreaks [Webinar training course]. Institute for Disaster Mental Health at SUNY New Paltz and New York Learns Public Health. Presented 2017 Jan 27. [Cited 2019 Jan 11]. Available from: https://www.urmc.rochester.edu/MediaLibraries/URMCMedia/flrtc/documents/Slides-MH-CONSEQUENCES-OF-ID-OUTBREAKSV2.pdf
8. Chen CS, Wu HY, Yang P, Yen CF. Psychological distress of nurses in Taiwan who worked during the outbreak of SARS. Psychiatr Serv. 2005;56(1):76–9.
9. Lee AM, Wong JGWS, McAlonan GM, Cheung V, Cheung C, Sham PC, et al. Stress and psychological distress among SARS survivors 1 year after the outbreak. Can J Psychiatr. 2007;52:233–40.

10. Styra R, Hawryluck L, Robinson S, Kasapinovic S, Fones C, Gold WL. Impact on health care workers employed in high-risk areas during the Toronto SARS outbreak. J Psychosom Res. 2008;64:177–83.
11. Chan AO, Huak CY. Psychological impact of the 2003 severe acute respiratory syndrome outbreak on health care workers in a medium size regional general hospital in Singapore. Occup Med (Lond). 2004;54:190–6. https://doi.org/10.1093/occmed/kqh027.
12. McAlonan GM, Lee AM, Cheung V, Cheung C, Tsang KW, Sham PC, et al. Immediate and sustained psychological impact of an emerging infectious disease outbreak on health care workers. Can J Psychiatr. 2007;52(4):241–7.
13. Qureshi DK, Gershon MRRM, Sherman MMF, Straub MT, Gebbie ME, McCollum MM, et al. Health care workers' ability and willingness to report to duty during catastrophic disasters. J Urban Heal. 2005;82:378–88.
14. Levin PJ, Gebbie EN, Qureshi K. Can the health-care system meet the challenge of pandemic flu? Planning, ethical, and workforce considerations. Public Health Rep. 2007;122(5):573–8.
15. Chan AO, Huak CY. Psychological impact of the 2003 severe acute respiratory syndrome outbreak on health care workers in a medium size regional general hospital in Singapore. Occup Med (Lond). 2004;54:190–6. https://doi.org/10.1093/occmed/kqh027.
16. Yap YG, Camm AJ. Drug induced QT prolongation and torsades de pointes. Heart. 2003;89(11):1363–72.
17. Yanofski J, Croarkin P. Choosing antidepressants for HIV and AIDS patients: insights on safety and side effects. Psychiatry (Edgmont). 2008;5(5):61–6.
18. Dubovsky AN, Arvikar S, Stern TA, Axelrod L. The neuropsychiatric complications of glucocorticoid use: Steroid psychosis revisited. Psychosomatics. 2012;53:103–15.

Chapter 12
Mental Health Assistance to Families and Communities in the Aftermath of an Outbreak

Jacqueline Levin

In the aftermath of a pandemic, family members of the afflicted both surviving and deceased will also require psychiatric support and care. For families whose loved ones have survived the illness, stressors will center around reintegrating into the family unit those patients who may be left with residual deficits and disabilities. For the bereaved families of those who perish in the pandemic, grief reactions are to be expected and may precipitate or worsen existing psychiatric disorders.

Grief reactions are variable with symptoms that are unique to the loss experienced, influenced by individual, social, religious, and cultural factors. Most often, symptoms are related to separation from the deceased (i.e., a yearning to be near, loneliness, and crying) or to stress and trauma (i.e., disbelief, shock, and numbness) [1]. Acute grief reactions are painful and impairing, but do not represent a mental illness.

J. Levin (✉)
Department of Psychiatry, North Shore University Hospital, Manhasset, NY, USA

© Springer Nature Switzerland AG 2019   143
D. Huremović (ed.), *Psychiatry of Pandemics*,
https://doi.org/10.1007/978-3-030-15346-5_12

Complicated grief reactions may also occur which are marked by maladaptive thoughts, feelings, and behaviors and can cause grief to become more intense and disabling. These individuals are best treated with cognitive behavioral therapy adapted for complicated grief [2].

Grief and loss counseling should be provided to the bereaved family members. Given a large number of human losses suffered during pandemics, bereavement support groups for surviving relatives will also play a therapeutic role on a larger scale and enhance a sense of social support, assuming family members are amenable to a group modality. Pharmacologic interventions in those instances center around treating distressing symptoms rather than bereavement itself (as bereavement is not a psychiatric illness). Anxiety and panic may be treated with benzodiazepines, for example, lorazepam 0.5–1 mg orally every 6 hours as needed. Insomnia may be treated with trazodone 25–100 mg orally at bedtime, melatonin 3 mg orally at bedtime, or with sedative-hypnotics. If a diagnosis of major depressive disorder is made in the course of bereavement, standard treatment with antidepressants is indicated.

Bereaved family members and loved ones of the deceased may also experience intense survivor's guilt which may manifest as dysphoria or questioning the meaning of life and why they were spared when their loved one was lost. Attending support groups, seeing a trusted mentor or spiritual leader, or seeking support from a therapist can help such individuals feel understood. A therapist can help challenge thought distortions contributing to guilt, and painful feelings can be processed [3].

Families should be educated on the importance of self-care which involves rest, nutritious diet, soothing activities, and regular exercise. Mental health providers should also aim to foster a sense of resilience in surviving family members. Resilience allows people to adapt well in the face of adversity and trauma while tolerating their pain and distress and can be developed through a number of strategies. Encouraging interconnectedness within and between surviving families can foster resilience by allowing for mutual help and support. Crises should not be viewed as insurmountable but rather as challenges that may be overcome. Change should be accepted as an inevitable part of life. Realistic goals and action plans should be established. Nurturing a positive self-image, maintaining hope, and keeping things in perspective can also help nurture resilience [4].

Other considerations in providing mental health care to surviving family members center around helping families obtain closure. It is important to remember that public health regulations in areas devastated by pandemics may outlaw traditional and religious burial rites. Communities experiencing mass fatalities will have to deal with the management of bodies; community leaders should collaborate with public health officials to guide surviving families on what should be done with the remains of their loved ones and, if known, how long the infectious agent remains in the deceased [5]. Spiritual leaders will play a critical role in keeping abreast of various religious rites of burial and can be helpful in liaising with the families of the deceased. It may also be helpful in these situations to provide families with photographs of their loved ones' bodies if physical access is not permitted [6]. In some cases, when communities have not been sensitive to these needs, family members have harbored their relatives at home and performed secret burials, becoming infected while preparing bodies of deceased loved ones [7].

It is important to note that just as survivors of pandemics may experience social stigma from their surrounding community, their family members, too, may be enshrouded by stigma. Friends may no longer want to visit the homes of the deceased for fear of contracting the disease, which promulgates further isolation. People may experience a loss or disruption of employment and experience financial hardships which will affect families, as well as experiencing scarcity of basic necessities such as food and water. Schools and daycares may have delayed reopenings or become permanently closed. In fact, the very fabric of a family may be irrevocably altered by human loss: loss of previous social supports, loss of caretakers for dependent family members, and loss of parents of children who are left orphaned by the disease. Mental health providers should be aware of and sensitive to the needs of changed and broken families, providing empathy and support as families struggle to adjust to their new realities. Children should also be given special consideration, reminding their caregivers to limit their exposure to traumatic news stories and to only give them age-appropriate information. Messages to older children should be targeted through schools, youth centers, and religious organizations [8].

Once the needs of patient's families are addressed in the aftermath of a pandemic, the question remains of how to address their greater communities at large and support them in the process of recovery and healing. In the face of tremendous adversity, communities can either rupture under relentless suffering, or they may band together in adaptive and prosocial ways to face the challenges that meet them. Just as the resilience of individuals can be nurtured, so can the resilience of communities. However, this is a task best initiated from the onset of a pandemic to help give people the resources they need to be courageous and unyielding.

Fundamental in containing public anxiety is a clear, transparent, and reliable system of communication. Frequent and accurate updates are the best way to reduce panic and rumors. Consistency is key from multiple trusted and expert sources; otherwise, people will develop a mistrust of the messages they receive, contributing to a sense of panic and erratic compliance with public health dictates. Consistent messages from multiple sources will increase the likelihood that the public will follow directions given by public health officials to reduce contagion [9]. A well-staffed hotline should be implemented and its number widely distributed by the media. Its staff should receive consistent messages and information to share with the public and should be equipped to handle the questions and concerns of callers. Specific time frames should be publicly shared for the next communication or announcement, and these time frames should be diligently adhered to, as people will come to depend on them. Doing so will also serve a symbolic purpose in fostering trust in the community that their leadership is reliable, accessible, and attuned to their needs. Communications should be translated to the local languages and dialects of at-risk communities, and staff members should be trained in cultural competence (bilingual and bicultural staff would be best). Multiple modalities should be used to distribute information to reach the broadest audience: television, telephone, text messages, radio, websites, podcasts, hotlines, pamphlets, and fact sheets [8].

From the outset of the pandemic, the public should be reminded of reasonable measures of protection with detailed information on precautions they can take. For example, it will be helpful to inform them of specific emergency kits and supplies to obtain; preparatory acts to improve access to these resources are prudent. People should be reminded to keep basic disaster supplies such as food, water, medications, first aid supplies, clothing, blankets, sanitation supplies, tools, flashlights, candles, can openers, batteries, baby supplies, and pet food, among others [8].

At-risk subpopulations should be identified and given additional information, or to their caregivers in the case of children. The elderly and medically compromised should be considered; it is helpful to collaborate with their primary care physicians to ensure they have access to several months' supply of necessary prescription medications and other myriad medical supplies in advance of the pandemic, in the event of shortages or impeded access. It may also be helpful to distribute information to the geriatric population through their senior centers and nursing homes. Special concerns for children should be considered, and information should be disseminated to parents, pediatricians, teachers, and daycare providers including ages affected, signs and symptoms, medical treatments indicated, as well as risk reduction strategies [8].

Psychological responses to community containment strategies (such as quarantine, social distancing, movement restrictions, school/work/other community closures) should be anticipated and planned for. Specific mental health challenges associated with quarantine and isolation are discussed separately in Chapter on Mental Health of Quarantine and Isolation. Voluntary social distancing measures may be requested of the community, existing on a spectrum ranging from maintaining a three-foot distance and avoiding physical contact to advising people to stay home and avoid public places. Travel restrictions may be imposed, and businesses may temporarily close or ask people to work from home. Schools, churches, and community centers may also be asked to temporarily suspend services and programs [8]. During these times, virtual contact via the internet, telephone, television, and radio should be promoted to decrease distressing feelings of isolation and frustration [5]. It is important to acknowledge and validate the disruption in routine and to thank the public for banding together to maintain the safety of the community for the greater good. Providing financial relief due to lost time/income from job closures may be quite helpful in reducing anxiety for those living in impoverished areas. Broadcasting online classwork through web-based programs can help reduce the disruption to students. Religious communities may choose to engage in virtual or online prayer groups and bible study.

Community mental health surveillance is critical as the pandemic subsides. Previous pandemics have shown that the absence of mental health and psychosocial support systems and a dearth of well-trained mental health professionals in affected countries have amplified the risks of enduring psychological distress and progression to psychopathology [7]. As public needs are being anticipated by community leaders, prior experiences have proven it is critical to fortify mental health resources and access. For example, providing educational materials informing the public of typical stress reactions can help normalize reactions and emphasize hope, resilience, and recovery [5]. Public mental health surveillance should be conducted in tandem with disease surveillance, addressing PTSD, depression, and substance use disorders. Recommendations should be provided for positive coping strategies, for example, by maintaining an updated website describing warning signs of pandemic-related mental health issues. Social media may play a useful role in helping to share and disseminate resources [10]. Meeting the psychosocial needs of the public (i.e., housing, transportation, schools, employment) and addressing the loss of critical infrastructure necessary to sustaining community function can help mitigate panic reactions [5].

Just as individuals and their families experience stigma associated with infection, quarantine, and survival, sometimes stigma can happen to entire communities. Community leaders should be attuned to pre-existing social conflicts during the pandemic, as these conflicts may later breed discrimination and marginalization. The stigma surrounding the illness can lead to the isolation of entire groups, impeding the recovery of the community in general [5]. In the aftermath of a pandemic, some members of the community might experience a loss of faith in their health institutions, employers, or government leaders. They may believe that medical resources have not been fairly distributed [11]. It is important in these moments to be mindful of the legacy of mistrust and negative beliefs left behind by the pandemic, for ignoring these beliefs can lead to alienation, despair, and further stigmatization.

Public memorials to honor the memory and sacrifice of the deceased may provide a pivotal role in reducing stigmatization and reframing the pandemic as a societal tragedy rather than one belonging to only certain groups or individuals. Community recognition and appreciation rituals such as speeches, memorial services, collection campaigns, and television specials are important tools for coping with community-wide loss and grief [5]. Events promoting social cohesion and unity, volunteer activities, and anniversary events can assist individuals and communities to move forward in their recovery [10].

Spiritual concerns of the community should also be addressed both during and after a pandemic. Community leaders should create partnerships with faith-based congregations and organizations at the onset of a pandemic, as religious leaders may be instrumental in liaising between the community and individuals whose religious or cultural beliefs (toward health care or burial rituals, for example) may put them at increased risk of harm. In the aftermath of a pandemic, spiritual events can help restore the fabric of the community and provide unique comfort and support to the bereaved during the grief and mourning. When congregations are finally able to meet again, their reunions should be jubilated and programs supporting recovery should be planned and celebrated [10]. If multiple congregations have suffered extensive human losses of their members, they may choose to band together to form new congregations and build anew; in these cases, they will serve as exemplars of the tenacity of the human spirit, not only for their congregants, but for the greater community at large.

References:

1. Shear MK, Reynolds III CF, Simon NM, Zisook S, Stein MB. Complicated grief in adults: Treatment. Post TW, editor. UpToDate. Waltham: UpToDate Inc. http://www.uptodate.com. Accessed 16 Dec 2018.
2. Shear MK, Reynolds III CF, Simon NM, Zisook S, Stein MB. Grief and bereavement in adults: clinical features. Post TW, editor. UpToDate. Waltham: UpToDate Inc. http://www.uptodate.com. Accessed 16 Dec 2018.
3. Good Therapy. Survivor guilt [Internet]. 2018 Jan 19 [cited 2019 Jan 11]. Available from: https://www.goodtherapy.org/blog/psychpedia/survivor-guilt
4. Comas-Diaz L, Luthar SS, Maddi SR, O'Neill HK, Saakvitne KW, Tedeschi RG. The road to resilience [internet brochure]. Washington, DC: American Psychological Association; [cited 2019 Jan 12]. Available from: http://www.apa.org/helpcenter/road-resilience.aspx
5. American Public Health Association. Preparing for pandemic influenza. Policy statement #20063 [internet]. Washington, DC: American Public Health Association; 2006 Nov 8 [cited 2019 Jan 12]. Available from: https://www.apha.org/policies-and-advocacy/public-health-policy-statements/policy-database/2014/07/18/09/19/preparing-for-pandemic-influenza
6. Reardon S. Ebola's mental-health wounds linger in Africa. Nature. 2015;519:13–4.
7. Shultz JM, Baingana F, Neria Y. The 2014 Ebola outbreak and mental health: current status and recommended response. JAMA. 2015;313(6):567–8.

8. Havice-Cover PJ, Drennen C. Pandemic influenza: quarantine, isolation and social distancing [Internet]. Colorado: The Colorado Department of Human Services Division of Mental Health. Available from: http://www.realisticpreparedness.com/downloads/PanFluQuarantineIsolation.pdf

9. Levin PJ, Gebbie EN, Qureshi K. Can the health-care system meet the challenge of pandemic flu? Planning, ethical, and workforce considerations. Public Health Rep. 2007;122(5):573–8.

10. Missouri Department of Health and Senior Services. Pandemic influenza plan: psychosocial services preparedness [Internet]. 2018 Sept. [Cited 2019 Jan 11]. Available from: https://health.mo.gov/emergencies/panflu/pdf/panfluplanpsychosocial.pdf

11. Shultz JM. Mental health consequences of infectious disease outbreaks. [Webinar training course]. Institute for Disaster Mental Health at SUNY New Paltz and New York Learns Public Health. Presented 2017 Jan 27. [Cited 2019 Jan 11]. Available from: https://www.urmc.rochester.edu/MediaLibraries/URMCMedia/flrtc/documents/Slides-MH-CONSEQUENCES-OF-ID-OUTBREAKSV2.pdf

Chapter 13
Immunization and Vaccination

Saira Hussain

Vaccination is considered to be one of the greatest achievements of public health and is the most effective method of preventing infectious diseases. Global vaccination programs have contributed to a decline in mortality and morbidity of various diseases. Widespread immunity due to vaccination is largely responsible for the eradication of smallpox the restriction of polio measles tetanus and many other diseases. The effectiveness of vaccination has been widely studied and verified for example the influenza vaccine the HPV vaccine and the chicken pox vaccine. The World Health Organization (WHO) reports that vaccines are currently available for 25 different preventable infections [1].

The terms *vaccine* and *vaccination* are derived from Variolae vaccinae (smallpox of the cow), the term devised by Edward Jenner to denote cowpox. He used this term in 1798 in the title of his Inquiry into the *Variolae vaccinae know as the Cow Pox*, in which he described the protective effect of cowpox against smallpox [2].

S. Hussain (✉)
Department of Psychiatry, North Shore University Hospital, Manhasset, NY, USA
e-mail: shussai1@northwell.edu

© Springer Nature Switzerland AG 2019
D. Huremović (ed.), *Psychiatry of Pandemics*,
https://doi.org/10.1007/978-3-030-15346-5_13

Sometime during the late 1760s, while serving his apprenticeship as a surgeon/apothecary, Edward Jenner learned of the story, common in rural areas, that dairy workers would never have the often-fatal or disfiguring disease smallpox, because they had already had cowpox, which has a very mild effect in humans. In 1796, Jenner took pus from the hand of a milkmaid with cowpox, scratched it into the arm of an 8-year-old boy, and 6 weeks later inoculated the boy with smallpox, afterward observing that he did not catch smallpox [3, 4]. Jenner extended his studies and in 1798 reported that his vaccine was safe in children and adults and could be transferred from arm-to-arm reducing reliance on uncertain supplies from infected cows [2].

In 1881, to honor Jenner, Louis Pasteur proposed that the terms should be extended to cover the new protective and safe inoculations being developed at the time. Prior to the introduction of relatively safe vaccination with material from cases of cowpox, smallpox could be prevented by deliberate inoculation of smallpox virus, a far more dangerous method known as variolation. The second generation of vaccines was introduced in the 1880s by Louis Pasteur who developed vaccines for chicken cholera and anthrax, [5] and from the late nineteenth century on, vaccines were considered a matter of national prestige, and first compulsory vaccination laws were passed.

The twentieth century saw the introduction of several successful vaccines, including those against diphtheria, measles, mumps, and rubella. Major achievements included the development of the polio vaccine in the 1950s and the eradication of smallpox during the 1960s and 1970s. As vaccines became more common, many people began taking them for granted. However, vaccines remain elusive for many important diseases, including herpes simplex, malaria, gonorrhea, and HIV.

There are different types of vaccines that have been developed and used in the community. Some of the types include inactivated, attenuated, toxoid, subunit, and conjugate vaccines. Inactivated vaccines contain inactivated, but previously virulent organisms that have been destroyed by chemicals, heat, or radiation [6]. Examples include the polio vaccine, hepatitis A, and rabies. Attenuated vaccines contain live, active viruses that have been cultivated under conditions that disable their virulent properties, or use closely related but less dangerous antigens to produce a broad immune response. Examples include yellow fever, measles, mumps, rubella, and typhoid. Toxoid vaccines are made from inactivated toxic compounds that cause illness rather than the microorganism. Examples include tetanus and diphtheria. Protein subunit vaccines contain fragments of the inactivated or attenuated microorganism to create an immune response, and these include hepatitis B, HPV.

The efficacy of a vaccine is dependent on a number of factors including the disease itself, the strain of vaccine, whether the vaccination schedule has been properly observed. Assorted factors such as ethnicity, age, and genetic predisposition play a role as well. In 1958, there were 763, 094 cases of measles in the United States; 552 deaths resulted [7]. After the introduction of new vaccines, the number of cases dropped to fewer than 150 per year [8]. In early 2008, there were 64 suspected cases of measles. Fifty-four of those infections were associated with importation from another country, although only 13% were actually acquired outside the United States; 63 of the 64 individuals either had been vaccinated against measles or were uncertain whether they had been vaccinated [8].

As long as the majority of people are vaccinated, it is much more difficult for an outbreak of disease to occur, let alone spread. This effect is called *herd immunity*. Polio, which is transmitted only between humans, is targeted by an extensive eradication campaign that has seen endemic polio restricted to only parts of three countries—Afghanistan, Nigeria, and Pakistan [8].

Vaccines also prevent the development of antibiotic resistance. For example, by greatly reducing the incidence of pneumonia caused by Streptococcus pneumonia, vaccine programs have greatly reduced the prevalence of infections resistant to penicillin or other first-line antibiotics [9].

Vaccinations given during childhood are generally safe [10]. Adverse effects, if any, are mostly mild. The rate of side effects depends on the vaccine in question. Some common side effects include fever, pain around the injection site, and muscle aches [11]. Some individuals may be allergic to particular ingredients in the vaccine. Severe side effects are, however, extremely rare. Varicella vaccine is rarely associated with complications in immunodeficient people and rotavirus vaccines are moderately associated with intussusception [10].

In order to provide the best protection, children are recommended to receive vaccinations as soon as their immune systems are sufficiently developed to respond to particular vaccines, with additional booster shots often required to achieve "full immunity". This, in turn, has led to the development of complex vaccination schedules. In the United States, the Advisory Committee on Immunization Practices, which recommends schedule additions for the Centers of Disease Control and Prevention, recommends routine vaccination of children against hepatitis A, hepatitis B, polio, mumps, measles, rubella, diphtheria, pertussis, tetanus, HiB, chickenpox, rotavirus, influenza, meningococcal disease, and pneumonia [12]. A large number of vaccines and boosters recommended (up to 24 injections by age 2) have led to problems with achieving full compliance. Various notification systems have been instituted and a number of combination injections are now marketed (e.g., pneumococcal conjugate vaccine and MMRV vaccine) to simplify schedule and improve compliance. Besides recommendations for infant vaccinations and boosters, many specific vaccines are recommended for other ages or for repeated injections throughout life—most commonly for measles, tetanus, influenza, and pneumonia. Pregnant women are often screened for continued resistance to rubella. The human papillomavirus vaccine is recommended in the United States (as of 2011) [13] and the United Kingdom (as of 2009) [14]. Vaccine recommendations for the elderly concentrate on pneumonia and influenza, which are more deadly to that group. Other countries may have vaccines in place to address diseases endemic to that area.

The principal challenge in further vaccine development is economic. Many of the diseases most demanding a vaccine, including HIV, malaria, and tuberculosis, exist principally in poor countries. Pharmaceutical firms and biotechnology companies have little incentive to develop vaccines for these diseases, because there is little revenue potential. Even in more affluent countries, financial returns are usually minimal, and the financial and other risks are great. Most vaccine development to date has relied on "push" funding by government, universities, and nonprofit organizations [15]. Many vaccines have been highly cost-effective and beneficial for public health. The number of vaccines actually administered has risen dramatically in recent decades. This increase, particularly in the number of different vaccines administered to children before entry into schools, may be due to government mandates and support, rather than an economic incentive.

Many vaccines need preservatives to prevent serious adverse effects such as *Staphylococcus* infection, which in one 1928 incident killed 12 of 21 children inoculated with a diphtheria vaccine that lacked a preservative [16]. Several preservatives are available, including thimerosal, phenoxyethanol, and formaldehyde. Thimerosal is more effective against bacteria, has a better shelf-life, and improves vaccine stability, potency, and safety; but, in the United States, the European Union, and a few other affluent countries, it is no longer used as a preservative in childhood vaccines, as a precautionary measure due to its mercury content [17]. Although controversial claims have been made that thimerosal contributes to autism, no convincing scientific evidence supports these claims [18].

The development of new delivery systems raises the hope of vaccines that are safer and more efficient to deliver and administer. Lines of research include liposomes and *ISCOM* (immune-stimulating complex) [19]. Other notable developments in vaccine delivery technologies have included oral vaccines. An oral polio vaccine, for example, turned out to be effective even when vaccinations were administered by volunteer staff without formal training; the results also demonstrated increased ease and efficiency of administering the vaccines. Effective oral vaccines have many advantages; for example, there is no risk of blood contamination. Vaccines intended for oral administration need not be liquid, and as solids, they commonly are more stable and less prone to damage or to spoilage by freezing in transport and storage [20]. Other promising, simplified approaches uses microneedles or needle-free delivery via patches [21, 22].

Vaccination policy is another critical element in attaining immunity at the international or global level. Such policies are mostly prerogatives of national authorities and can vary across the world. Some international agencies such as WHO or EU also affect the immunization agenda. In the European Union, for example, The European Commission assists member countries with the coordination of policies and programs and, in April 2018, it proposed a Council Recommendation to strengthen the EU cooperation on vaccine-preventable diseases. The initiative aims to tackle vaccine hesitancy, improve coordination on vaccine procurement, support research and innovation, and strengthen EU cooperation on vaccine-preventable diseases.

EU countries are encouraged to develop and implement national vaccination plans with initiatives to improve coverage and to introduce routine vaccination status checks. In addition, the Commission supports EU countries in maintaining or increasing rates of vaccination by promoting seasonal flu vaccination to at-risk groups. Though European vaccination rates are high overall, measles continues to spread where vaccination rates have declined, the World Health Organization warned in 2016.

In the United States, there is a similar program, with individual states creating their own individual schedules and requirements, and federal bodies, such as CDC, providing recommendations and guidelines. In the rest of the world, similarly, many countries rely on the guidelines and recommendations provided by the WHO, but are free to set their schedules and regulate immunizations as they see fit.

Vaccination in the Context of a Pandemic Outbreak

Vaccination, if available, will likely be a principal part of multifaceted public health response to the future emergence of a pandemic illness. In addition to other measures designed to respond to and control a pandemic, such as surveillance, communication plans, quarantine, and disease treatment, the deployment of effective vaccines has the biggest potential to protect lives and limit disease spread. Not all disease threats, however, have a corresponding vaccine, and for those that do, there are significant challenges to their successful use in a pandemic.

In the case of influenza viruses, for example, existing vaccines may not be effective against new strains. Though production methods and infrastructure for influenza vaccines are well established, each new influenza strain requires a new vaccine. Thus, any new pandemic influenza vaccine will take about 4–6 months to produce in large quantities [23]. For other newly emerging threats without licensed vaccines, such as SARS, Marburg virus, Nipah virus, and the like, the time required to develop and produce a safe, effective vaccine is unknown and would depend on the nature of the threat and the state of current vaccine research for that threat. In almost all cases, several months would be needed to respond with the first doses of vaccines. Until a safe, effective vaccine was ready, other public health and medical measures, such as social distancing, quarantine, and use of antiviral medications, would need to be employed to try to limit disease spread.

A variety of US federal, state, and local agencies are involved in public health emergency preparedness and response. The US Congress funds the Centers for Disease Control and Preventions Office of Public Health Preparedness and Response (PHPR) to build and strengthen national preparedness for public health emergencies caused by natural, accidental, or intentional events. Part of the CDC's funding supports the Strategic National Stockpile, which manages stores of vaccines and drugs that may be deployed in national emergencies.

The US Department of Health and Human Services (HHS) includes several offices involved in pandemic and bioterror response. The Office of the Assistant Secretary for Preparedness and Response (ASPR) was created after Hurricane Katrina and is responsible for leadership in prevention, preparation, and response to the adverse health effects of public health emergencies and disasters. ASPR conducts research and builds federal emergency medical operational capabilities. Within ASPR, the Biomedical Advanced Research and Development Authority (BARDA) is responsible for the development and purchase of the necessary vaccines, drugs, therapies, and diagnostic tools for public health medical emergencies [24].

State and local health departments, as well as public and private hospitals and local law enforcement agencies, would also be involved in responding to a pandemic public health emergency. Their roles are outlined in national response plans as well as delineated by organization-specific plans. The US FDA is involved in establishing a research agenda pandemic response, and it controls the pathway to licensure for vaccines, treatments, diagnostic tests, and other tools for responding to biological threats. The regulatory requirements for the licensure of a vaccine are complex and apply to a multistep process of safety, immunogenicity, efficacy testing, and post-licensure surveillance [24].

In situations when a new vaccine is needed quickly, the FDA has developed alternative pathways to licensure. One is an accelerated pathway to approval that might apply in the case of life-threatening disease when a new process will produce a vaccine with a meaningful therapeutic benefit over existing options. In other, more drastic threats, the so-called animal rule might be used—if research toward a vaccine or treatment would necessitate exposing humans to a toxic threat, then animal studies may be sufficient for approval. To date, these two rapid pathways have not been invoked for vaccines.

The US Emergency Use Authorization (EUA) is an option in pandemic response. After a declaration of emergency by the Department of Health and Human Services secretary, this program allows for use of an unapproved medical product (or a product that has been approved but not for the specific use applicable to the situation at hand) that is the best available treatment or prevention for the threat in question. EUAs were issued for antiviral treatments, a respirator, and a PCR diagnostic test during the 2009 A/H1N1 pandemic [25].

In all pandemic situations in which a vaccine is available or potentially available, a large supply of vaccine would be necessary and would be needed quickly. Currently, the US Strategic National Stockpile includes several types of influenza vaccines, including an H5N1 vaccine [26]. The stockpile also holds millions of doses of other vaccines, antibodies, antiviral medications, and other medical supplies. Should any of these stockpiled vaccines directly relate to an emerging pandemic, they would be deployed. Chances are, however, that an emerging pandemic illness will require a new vaccine and that will require time and resources to develop.

Another complicating factor to pandemic influenza vaccine production involves how the vaccine is made. Since the 1940s, seasonal and pandemic influenza vaccines have been produced in chicken eggs. The virus is introduced in the allantoic fluid of the fertilized egg (this is the fluid that bathes the embryo and yolk sac), and it replicates in the membrane surrounding the fluid. After about 3 days, the virus-containing fluid is harvested from each egg and the rest of the manufacturing process proceeds [27]. Dependence on egg-based vaccine production is, however, problematic even with non-pandemic seasonal influenza vaccine. First, eggs must be available in large quantities when vaccine production is to begin. Any disruption in egg supply—such as disease affecting chickens, or bad weather interfering with the shipping of eggs—can mean a delay in vaccine production. Second, some influenza strains grow more slowly or less robustly than others, which can result in delays or in lower yields of vaccine virus from each egg. Third, it is possible that some viral vaccine strains, given the origin of some influenza viruses in birds, may be toxic to eggs. In that case, egg-based influenza vaccine production methods would be useless. Even under the best of circumstances, the influenza vaccine production can provide vaccines for less than half the global population.

Other promising technologies are being explored for the development of a universal influenza vaccine, which is the ultimate goal for many influenza vaccine programs, and would serve as a paragon for any future pandemic. Such a vaccine might need to be given only once, rather than every year as with current seasonal vaccines. Such a universal vaccine would ideally provide protection against all, or at least most, of the many strains of influenza capable of making people sick, including future pandemic influenzas. Plant-produced influenza vaccines are in clinical trials and may prove to be a useful alternative to egg- and cell-based vaccines.

In the event of a pandemic, the public and private sectors will mobilize to produce and distribute the vaccine, if one is available, as quickly as possible. The CDC's Advisory Committee on Immunization Practices and other governmental and advisory groups will issue national guidelines prioritizing who should be vaccinated. State and local health departments will develop local modifications to the recommendations as needed. These public health departments will need to make decisions about how to distribute the vaccine to providers within their jurisdictions equitably and efficiently with the goal of reaching the priority groups first.

Methods for distributing the vaccine in a pandemic are outlined in the HHS Pandemic Influenza Plan, which details public sector pandemic response [28]. The plans are designed to provide guidance to public health coordinators, but also to be flexible enough to adapt to the unique conditions of the particular pandemic situation. For example, prior to the 2009 H1N1 pandemic, the most recent pandemic influenza emergency response plans had been based on H5N1 influenza. Planners accordingly projected that healthcare providers would be overwhelmed with caring for the sick and would not have the capacity to administer the vaccine. Distribution plans primarily relied on public entities, such as public health departments and hospitals, to receive the vaccine and vaccinate most of the targeted population. But because 2009 H1N1 influenza did not cause such severe disease, public health authorities realized early on that providers would have the capacity to vaccinate patients. And so vaccine was, for the most part, shipped directly to providers based on the distribution system for the federal Vaccines for Children (VFC) program. This required a few changes to usual VFC procedures, most notably to include non-VFC providers, such as retail pharmacies, corporations with occupational health clinics, and non-pediatric healthcare providers, that received and administered vaccines.

Most aspects of vaccine distribution were executed smoothly in the 2009 H1N1 pandemic, especially considering that limited supplies of vaccines had to be allocated fairly and that initial demand was high [29]. The role of certain private vaccine providers attracted media attention and raised some public concern, especially when a few large high-profile private employers received the vaccine before some public entities did. No wrongdoing was alleged, but the situation drew attention to the mechanism of vaccine distribution when a variety of public and private provider types are included. However, public health authorities support the use of private occupational health clinics to vaccinate in a pandemic, since they are able to identify and reach many people in high-priority groups.

Reports by state health departments after the pandemic assessing the H1N1 vaccination program suggest a few areas of improvement in a future pandemic: two issues that surfaced frequently in the reports were the need for accurate supply forecasts to inform vaccine ordering and subsequent distribution, as well as the need for clear communication about priority groups for vaccination [30].

The US federal government conducts periodic simulations of biologic emergencies to assess the effectiveness of the public health response and to identify areas where response needs to be improved.

The European Union currently has a tool to respond to pandemic influenza threats that the United States has not yet employed. Oil-in-water adjuvants have been used in the influenza vaccine in the European Union since 1997 and have an established safety record. But, while plans were made to use adjuvant in the US 2009 H1N1 vaccine, authorities abandoned those and instead approved only unadjuvanted vaccines. Even if the adjuvanted influenza vaccine were released, the US public might be reluctant to take the unfamiliar vaccine, in spite of its safety record in the EU.

Vaccine acquisition, distribution, and uptake issues are substantially different in the developing world. Less wealthy countries typically do not widely use influenza vaccine for a variety of reasons, perhaps the most prominent of which is the need to devote health funds to more pressing concerns. In the event of a deadly influenza pandemic or other disease outbreak requiring mass vaccination, governments of developing countries will face significant challenges such as meeting supply needs, funding vaccine acquisition and ensuring uptake of vaccine in places where influenza vaccination is not commonly practiced.

Under the guidance of the World Health Organization and with the support of various governments, many middle-income and developing countries (Brazil, Egypt, India, Indonesia, Iran, Mexico, Republic of Korea, Romania, Serbia, Thailand, and Viet Nam) have established influenza vaccine manufacturing capacity, or are making progress to develop this capacity. The US and Japanese governments have funded influenza vaccine manufacturing capacity in several countries in Latin America and Asia in an attempt to build readiness in the event of an influenza pandemic. Efforts will help to establish seasonal influenza vaccine production that could then be harnessed in an influenza pandemic. WHO officials note that global seasonal influenza capacity has increased from 350 million doses in 2006 to more than 800 million doses in 2011. Because the seasonal vaccine is trivalent (that is, it includes three strains of influenza virus), pandemic vaccine capacity should be roughly triple that of seasonal influenza capacity—2.4 billion doses. This is still far short of total global need, but it is evident that global influenza vaccine production capacity is increasing.

Mental Health Aspects of Immunization and Vaccination

Several claims about the neuropsychiatric adverse effects of vaccinations have been staked over the past two decades, stirring considerable public debate and affecting the immunization rates in some communities [31].

One evidence-based study where some temporal relationship was found was a pilot study, from Penn State and Yale University researchers, looking at medical private insurance claims in a large database and comparing children and adolescents aged 6–15 years prior year's vaccination records with the new diagnosis of a number of neuropsychiatric disorders over 5 years [32].

The temporal association was found for several diagnostic entities, the most relevant one for anorexia nervosa. Children who had been vaccinated within the prior 3 months had an 80% elevated risk of getting a new diagnosis of the eating disorder that has been increasing in recent years, compared to controls. Less pronounced association was found between vaccinations and OCD, tic disorders, and anxiety disorders.

Incidentally, in the control group, children with broken bones were also slightly more likely to have received the influenza vaccine during the previous year, but by a much smaller percentage. Curiously, children with major depression and bipolar disorder were *less* likely to have received the influenza vaccine, but again with smaller hazard ratios.

The researchers found correlations for one vaccine in particular: the influenza vaccine, which was associated with higher rates of OCD, anorexia, anxiety disorder, and tic disorder. The study emphasized that there was no "proof of a causal role" in vaccines for any of the conditions.

A biological explanation for these correlations has not been found, but a potential mechanism could lie in the body's immune response to vaccines, the study suggested. Cross-reactivity has been explored as one of the hypotheses providing a possible connection. Cross-reactivity occurs when vaccine-induced antibodies react against not only the intended pathogen proteins but also against human proteins. For example, a 2015 study published in Science Translational Medicine discovered that antibodies elicited by the pandemic influenza vaccine cross-reacted with a human brain protein — hypocretin receptor 2.

Autoimmunity, in which antibodies attack human proteins, occurs independently of immunization and also may play a role in normal brain development and in early-onset psychiatric disorders [33]. Some authors (Leckman) hypothesize that, if children were experiencing inflammation—a process that promotes autoimmunity—at the time of vaccination, the combination of inflammation and vaccination could have deleterious effects on brain development [34].

In modern society, any potentially serious adverse event attributed to vaccination is likely to be snapped up by the media, particularly newspapers and television, as it appeals to the emotions of the public. Thus, for example, considerable attention was devoted to the publication of Andrew Wakefield's article, which linked measles vaccination to pervasive developmental disorders and nonspecific colitis, [35] and to the case of Heather Whitestone, who was elected Miss America despite her deafness, which had erroneously been attributed to the diphtheria, tetanus, and pertussis vaccine [36]. The widespread news of the alleged adverse events of vaccination has helped to create the "urban myth" that vaccines cause serious neurological disorders and has boosted anti-vaccination associations. These movements and associations, however, are nothing new. They can be traced back to the nineteenth century, with the foundation of the National Anti-Vaccination League in 1896 in Britain and the Anti-Vaccination Society of America in 1879 in the United States were established. By the end of the twentieth century, opposition to vaccinations had strengthened in most developed countries because diseases preventable by vaccinations had become increasingly rare. Thus, with regard to the subject of vaccinations, ethical, social, religious, and legal issues cannot be ignored.

When Mumps/Measles/Rubella (MMR) vaccines are concerned, the *British Medical Journal* defined the main study that linked these vaccines to autism as a "deliberate fraud" [37]. This conclusion resulted from an investigation conducted by the investigative journalist Brian Deer into the research originally published in 1998 by the journal the

Lancet, before being withdrawn in February 2010. The paper had associated the administration of MMR vaccine with a new syndrome characterized by autism and ileal lymphoid hyperplasia associated with nonspecific colitis. According to Fiona Godlee, the editor in chief of the BMJ, the article by Wakefield "was based not on bad science but on a deliberate fraud". The US Institute of Medicine (IOM) also concluded that "The evidence favors rejection of a causal relationship between MMR vaccine and autism" [38].

When the relationship between vaccines and schizophrenia is concerned, no epidemiological studies have shown the existence of a causal link. In addition, Short et al. have demonstrated that babies born to rhesus monkeys infected with the flu virus during pregnancy have both significantly smaller brains than normal and other brain abnormalities seen in schizophrenia [39]. These results are consistent with the findings of Mednick et al. [40], who reported an increased risk of schizophrenia in persons who had been in the fetal stage in 1957—the time of the pandemic known as the "Asian" pandemic—and with the study by Byrne et al. [41] Vaccination should therefore be considered a valuable tool, particularly during pregnancy, in that it may also help reduce schizophrenia. Indeed, the CDC recommends influenza vaccination in any period of gestation.

Acceptance of vaccines is a major driver of uptake, along with issues of access, affordability, and awareness. In the past decade, parents have been questioning the need for and safety of vaccines, and as a result, vaccination rates have fallen to dangerously low levels in certain communities. The effects of vaccine hesitancy are widespread. Community pediatricians who interact regularly with vaccine-hesitant parents report a higher level of burnout and lower levels of job satisfaction. Vaccine hesitancy has been linked to increased emergency department use, morbidity, and mortality. Nonacceptance of vaccination is a phenomenon that concerns global agencies. In 2012, a World Health Organization (WHO), a working group, was formed to address vaccine hesitancy and its implications [42]. Vaccine hesitancy is best viewed on a spectrum of parental beliefs and concerns. From the perspective of medical providers, vaccine hesitancy is demonstrated by increased requests for alternative vaccinations schedules or by altogether postponing or declining vaccines. The percentage of parents who refuse all vaccines is small in comparison to alternative schedules.

Overall childhood vaccination rates remain relatively high in the United States. Rates of undervaccination in children younger than 2 continue to rise. In Oregon, for example, rates of alternative schedules have quadrupled. Poland and Jacobson point out that "since the 18th century, fear and mistrust have arisen every time a new vaccine has been introduced" [43]. Even amidst the deadly smallpox epidemic, increasing resistance to smallpox vaccine led to mandated vaccination in the United Kingdom. The United States dealt with its own opposition to mandatory smallpox vaccinations, eventually leading to Supreme Court Case Jacobsen v. Massachusetts, 197, U.S. 1 (1905).

There is a broad spectrum of individuals who choose not to have themselves or their children vaccinated. They are most commonly referred to as "vaxxers" or "vaccine deniers." These range from individuals who are solidly anti-vaccine, often termed "vaccine rejectors" (VRj), to those who may accept or even advocate for most vaccines but have concerns over 1 or more vaccines [44]. Hagood and Mintzer Herlihy suggested a 3-category model, characterizing individuals as vaccine rejectors (VRj), vaccine-resistant (VR), or vaccine-hesitant (VH) [45]. Vaccine rejectors are those who are "unyieldingly entrenched in their refusal to consider vaccine information," prone to conspiracy theory thinking, and may eschew traditional medical providers altogether in favor of "complementary" or "alternative" medical practices. The VRs are those who may currently reject vaccination but are still willing to consider information, and they have a lower incidence of belief in conspiracy theories than VRj individuals. The VH individuals tend to have anxiety about vaccinations but are not committed to vaccine refusal. These groups correspond roughly to the "refusers," "late/selective vaccinators," and "the hesitant." Interventions targeted at changing minds or attitudes to increase vaccine acceptance need to take into consideration the wide spectrum of beliefs regarding vaccines to be properly tailored to the individual, rather than assuming that all individuals with vaccine concerns have a single belief system.

The reasons for the increasing prevalence of vaccine hesitancy are numerous. Vaccines have become, as many have described, "victims of their own success." An article in *The Economist* further argues that "the risks of the vaccine are visible; its benefits are not" [46]. Vaccines have been seen as so highly effective and are no longer seen as necessary by many parents, because the diseases they prevent are virtually unknown to the general population. As rates of vaccine-preventable diseases dwindle, caregivers may grow to fear the vaccine more than the disease it prevents, thus leading to decreased vaccination rates [47].

Additionally, highly publicized anti-vaccine arguments have caused a tremendous public backlash against vaccines. The best-known argument originated in an article in *The Lancet*, in which Wakefield falsified data to establish a link between MMR vaccine and autism. Although the article was later retracted, and Wakefield's license was removed, the damage to the public was already done. There has been no shortage of celebrities, including Jenny McCarthy, Alicia Silverstone, Jim Carey, Kirstie Alley, and President Donald Trump who have expressed concern regarding vaccines, not directly opposing vaccines. As concerns for vaccines rise, there is growing popular interest in alternative remedies and products which has led many parents to question toxins in vaccines. Other parental concerns include multiple needlesticks, and too many vaccines for the immune system to handle [47].

Trust in institutional medicine has become lower than ever before, and medical providers' relationships with patients are changing. More parents have come to value and expect a shared decision-making model with their pediatrician. These cultural shifts have occurred in the context of a vaccine schedule that has become more crowded with a substantial increase in the number of vaccines given to a child before age 2 since 1994. Parental concerns regarding the number of vaccines received at a single visit is a well-documented reason for delaying or refusing vaccines [47].

The Internet has played a pivotal role in enhancing parental concerns over vaccines in the last decade as well. Even if parents attempt to educate themselves about the risks and benefits of vaccines, they are often left feeling confused and frustrated due to mixed messages presented on social media and Internet sources. The Internet is filled with blogs, websites, and articles touting the dangers of vaccines, leaving parents uncertain of which sources to trust. A search of the term *vaccination* on the Internet can lead to more anti-vaccination materials than pro-vaccination materials, and even returns cerfully crafted YouTube videos as the top query results [48].

The proportion of parents who are vaccine-hesitant varies substantially across the United States and geographic clustering of nonmedical vaccination exemptions has been well documented. Although this clustering effect is not entirely understood, one may hypothesize that the culture of a local population, influenced by characteristics such as socioeconomic status, race, ethnicity, and education level, may play a role. Data from the National Immunization Survey from 1995 to 2001 demonstrated that unvaccinated children were more likely to be white, to have a married, college-educated mother, to belong to higher income households, compared to undervaccinated children [47].

The well-publicized 2014–2015 Disneyland measles outbreak was a stark reminder of the direct influence of vaccine hesitancy and refusal. However, we have seen the influence over the decades in the United States. In a nationally representative survey, 48% of pediatricians and family doctors reported spending less than 10 minutes discussing vaccines with parents who had concerns about vaccines. Considering that the average well-child visit is 18 minutes long, families with concerns about vaccines are likely missing out on other anticipatory guidance [49].

Glanz et al. have done extensive work on direct risks of vaccine refusal on actual vaccination rates and the incidence of disease. Children whose parents refuse pertussis-containing vaccines are 23 times more likely to be diagnosed with pertussis, children whose parents refuse varicella vaccine are nine times more likely to be diagnosed with chicken pox, and children whose parents refused the pneumococcal vaccine are 6 times more likely to be hospitalized for invasive pneumococcal disease or lobar pneumonia. Numerous studies have shown that states and communities with higher rates of vaccine exemptions are more prone to outbreaks of vaccine-preventable diseases such as measles, mumps, and pertussis [50].

One of the factors that interrelate with individuals' vaccine rejection is the use of complementary and alternative medicine (CAM) Eve Dube et al. 2013. Katie Attwell et al. found with 20 parents who had refused or delayed some of or all of their children's vaccines had a "do it yourself ethic" and personal agency enhanced by CAM use [51]. These parents viewed vaccines as being toxic, profit motive, and embraced CAM as a protective strategy for immune systems before, during, and after an illness. Parents were inclined to pursue CAM care due to their upbringings, or recommendations from within their social community, where vaccine questioning was prominent. Parents or their children experienced specific health problems (not necessarily vaccine related), whereby Western Medicine was viewed "to hit a wall," and CAM filled the gap, generating questions about the vaccines. Parents who prefer CAM, an approach sometimes also euphemistically called "health-promoting" or "salutogenic," tend to cluster in certain parts of the United States, such as rural northern Idaho, or urban pockets of Seattle, Spokane, Portland in the Pacific Northwest, as well as some other urban regions in the country [52].

Immunization hesitancy can also be identified among some religiously conservative populations in the United States that turned out to be receptive audiences for anti-vaccine social media activists. In 2017, after being targeted with misinformation about vaccine risks which led to lower immunization rates, Somali-Minnesotan community experienced a measles outbreak [53]. In 2018, a small measles outbreak was recorded among children in Orthodox Jewish communities in and around New York City [54].

There have been extensive efforts to develop strategies to address vaccine-hesitant parents. To date, there are a few effective evidence-based strategies for communication with parents or for addressing vaccine hesitancy at the community level. There is robust literature showing that simply providing information often does not lead to people changing their views and may even create a dynamic in which a patient or parent is actually less receptive to information a provider may impart [55]. It is clear that medical providers play a crucial role in influencing parents' decision to vaccinate. A recent Cochrane Review revealed that parents wanted more, unbiased vaccine information than they had been receiving. The review also showed that poor communication and poor relationships with providers had the ability to negatively influence vaccine decisions. Building a trusting relationship with parents and patients can promote vaccine acceptance and also influence other important aspects of care [56].

To a rational healthcare provider, particularly in times of emergency, vaccine hesitancy may seem irrational and nonsensical. As irrational, and unfounded as it may be, it must not be dismissed. Failure to address vaccine hesitancy may as well translate into a catastrophic failure to immunize, even in times of dire need. It is a serious issue that needs to be addressed in a serious manner.

There is no single intervention strategy that addresses all instances of vaccine hesitancy. Based on the Systematic Review of Strategies to Address Vaccine Hesitancy, the most effective interventions addressing the outcome of vaccination uptake are multicomponent interventions versus single component. These interventions should be dialogue-based and directly targeted at the unvaccinated or undervaccinated populations [57].

The interventions should address the specific determinants underlying vaccine hesitancy, which may include the following:

- Engagement of religious or other influential leaders to promote vaccination in the community
- Social mobilization
- Improving convenience and access to vaccination
- Mandating vaccination/sanctions for non-vaccination

- Employing reminder and follow-up
- Communications training for HCW
- Non-financial incentives
- Aim to increase knowledge, awareness about vaccination

Motivational interviewing has been a particularly helpful approach with hesitant parents. Motivational interviewing is the process of engaging in open-ended discussion with an individual to assess an individual's readiness to change with the goal of drawing upon the person's own desire and motivation to change, rather than the provider's motivation. In the 2016 Clinical Report on Countering Vaccine Hesitancy by the American Academy of Pediatrics, motivational interviewing is listed as a potential communication technique that may be helpful as pediatricians discuss vaccines with hesitant parents [58]. In a recent cluster randomized trial, motivational interviewing was shown to be effective at increasing uptake of HPV vaccine [59].

Immunization hesitancy represents a considerable and growing obstacle toward achieving appropriate levels of immunization under everyday circumstances. It is virtually impossible to anticipate in what manner and to what extent immunization hesitancy would interfere with immunization rollout during a pandemic. In addition to paramount legal, ethical, and logistical challenges to mounting a response to a pandemic outbreak, immunization hesitancy may seem irrational, unnecessary, and capricious. In case of an outbreak, however, it will not be trivial, and anyone who fails to take it seriously will jeopardize any success in fighting a deadly pandemic outbreak.

References

1. World Health Organization. Global vaccine action plan 2011–2020. Geneva; 2012.
2. Baxby D. Edward Jenner's inquiry; a bicentenary analysis. Vaccine. 1999;17(4):301–7.

3. Stern AM, Markel H. The history of vaccines and immunization: familiar patterns, new challenges. Health Aff. 2005;24(3):611–21.
4. Dunn PM. Dr Edward Jenner (1749–1823) of Berkeley, and vaccination against smallpox. Arch Dis Child Fetal Neonatal Ed. 1996;74(1):F77–8.
5. Pasteur L. Address on the germ theory. Lancet. 1881;118(3024):271–2.
6. Sinha JK, Bhattacharya S. A text book of immunology (Google book preview). Academic Publishers. p. 318. ISBN 978-81-89781-09-5. Retrieved January 09, 2014.
7. Orenstein WA, Papania MJ, Wharton ME. Measles elimination in the United States. J Infect Dis. 2004;189(Suppl 1):S1–3.
8. Measles—United States, January 1 – April 25, 2008. Morb Mortal Wkly Rep. 2008;57(18):494–8.
9. Abbott A. Vaccines promoted as key to stamping out drug-resistant microbes. 2017 July 19. Immunization can stop resistant infections before they get started, say scientists from industry and academia.
10. Maglione MA, Das L, Raaen L, Smith A, Chari R, Newberry S, Shanman R, Perry T, Goetz MB, Gidengil C. Safety of vaccines used for routine immunization of US children: a systematic review. Pediatrics. 2014;134(2):325–37.
11. Possible Side-effects from Vaccines. Centers for disease control and prevention. Retrieved February 24, 2014.
12. ACIP Vaccine Recommendations Home Page. CDC. 2013 Nov 15. Retrieved January 10, 2014.
13. HPV Vaccine Safety. Centers for Disease Control and Prevention (CDC). 2013 Dec 20. Retrieved January 10, 2014.
14. HPV vaccine in the clear. NHS choices. 2009 Oct 02. Retrieved January 10, 2014.
15. Olesen OF, Lonnroth A, Mulligan B. Human vaccine research in the European Union. Vaccine. 2009;27(5):640–5.
16. Thimerosal in vaccines. Center for Biologics Evaluation and Research, U.S. Food and Drug Administration. 2007 Sept 06. Retrieved October 01, 2007.
17. Bigham M, Copes R. Thiomersal in vaccines: balancing the risk of adverse effects with the risk of vaccine-preventable disease. Drug Saf. 2005;28(2):89–101.
18. Offit PA. Thimerosal and vaccines—a cautionary tale. N Engl J Med. 2007;357(13):1278–9.
19. Morein B, Hu KF, Abusugra I. Current status and potential application of ISCOMs in veterinary medicine. Adv Drug Deliv Rev. 2004;56(10):1367–82.

20. Khan FA. Biotechnology fundamentals. CRC Press; 2011 Sept 20. p. 270. ISBN 9781439820094.
21. Giudice EL, Campbell JD. Needle-free vaccine delivery. Adv Drug Deliv Rev. 2006;58(1):68–89.
22. Australian scientists develop 'needle-free' vaccination. The Sydney Morning Herald. 2013 August 18.
23. http://www.who.int/csr/disease/swineflu/notes/ h1n1_vaccine_20090806/en/
24. https://www.historyofvaccines.org/content/articles/ vaccines-pandemic-threats
25. https://www.cdc.gov/h1n1flu/cdcresponse.htm
26. http://www.cidrap.umn.edu/news-perspective/2008/04/ hhs-adds-h5n1-clade-22-vaccine-stockpile
27. https://www.historyofvaccines.org/content/blog/ us-cell-line-facility-produce-pandemic-influenza-vaccine
28. https://www.cdc.gov/flu/pandemic-resources/planning-prepared-ness/national-strategy-planning.html
29. Huang H-C. Equalizing access to pandemic influenza vaccines through optimal allocation to public health distribution points. PLoS One. 2017;12(8):e0182720.
30. https://www.hsdl.org/?view&did=714799
31. Dubé E, Laberge C, Guay M, Bramadat P, Roy R, Bettinger J. Vaccine hesitancy: an overview. Hum Vaccin Immunother. 2013;9(8):1763–73.
32. Leslie DL, Kobre RA, Richmand BJ, Aktan Guloksuz S, Leckman JF. Temporal association of certain neuropsychiatric disorders following vaccination of children and adolescents: a pilot case–control study. Front Psych. 2017;8:3. https://doi.org/10.3389/fpsyt.20.
33. Raevuori A, Haukka J, Vaarala O, Suvisaari JM, Gissler M, Grainger M, et al. The increased risk for autoimmune diseases in patients with eating disorders. PLoS One. 2014;9(8):e104845. https://doi.org/10.1371/journal.pone.0104845.
34. Leckman JF, Vaccarino FM. Editorial commentary: "what does immunology have to do with brain development and neuro-psychiatric disorders?" Brain Res. 2015;1617:1–6. https://doi.org/10.1016/j.brainres.2014.09.052.
35. Wakefield AJ, Murch SH, Anthony A, Linnell J, Casson DM, Malik M, Berelowitz M, Dhillon AP, Thomson MA, Harvey P, Valentine A, Davies SE, Walker-Smith JA. Ileal-lymphoid-nodular hyperplasia, non-specific colitis, and pervasive develop-mental disorder in children. Lancet. 1998;351(9103):637–41.

36. Gasparini R, Panatto D, Lai PL, Amicizia D. The "urban myth" of the association between neurological disorders and vaccinations. J Prev Med Hyg. 2015;56(1):E1–8.

37. Godlee F, Smith J, Marcovitch H. Wakefield's article linking MMR vaccine and autism was fraudulent. BMJ. 2011;342:c7452.

38. IOM (Institute of Medicine). Adverse effects of vaccines: evidence and causality. Washington, DC: The National Academies Press; 2011.

39. Short SJ, Lubach GR, Karasin AI, Olsen CW, Styner M, Knickmeyer RC, Gilmore JH, et al. Maternal influenza infection during pregnancy impacts postnatal brain development in the rhesus monkey. Biol Psychiatry. 2010;6:965–73.

40. Mednick SA, Machon RA, Huttunen MO, et al. Adult schizophrenia following prenatal exposure to an influenza epidemic. Arch Gen Psychiatry. 1988;45:189–92.

41. Byrne M, Agerbo E, Bennedsen B, et al. Obstetric conditions and risk of first admission with schizophrenia: a Danish national register based study. Schizophr Res. 2007;97:51–9.

42. https://www.who.int/immunization/sage/meetings/2014/october/SAGE_working_group_revised_report_vaccine_hesitancy.pdf

43. Poland GA, Jacobson RM. The age-old struggle against the antivaccinationists. N Engl J Med. 2011;364(2):97–9. https://doi.org/10.1056/NEJMp1010594.

44. Tara CS. Vaccine rejection and hesitancy: a review and call to action. Open Forum Infect Dis. 2017;4(3). https://doi.org/10.1093/ofid/ofx146.

45. Hagood EA, Mintzer Herlihy S. Addressing heterogeneous parental concerns about vaccination with a multiple-source model: a parent and educator perspective. Hum Vaccin Immunother. 2013;9(8):1790–4.

46. The needle and the damage done. The Economist. 2002. http://www.economist.com/node/987833?zid=318&ah=ac379c09c1c3fb67e0e8fd1964d5247f. Accessed Oct 2018.

47. McClure CC, Cataldi J, T'Oleary S. Vaccine hesitancy, where we are and where we are going. Clin Ther. 2017;39:1550–62.

48. Wakefield MA, Loken B, Hornik RC. Use of mass media campaigns to change health behaviour. Lancet (London, England). 2010;376(9748):1261–71.

49. Kempe A, Daley MF, McCauley MM, Crane LA, Suh CA, Kennedy AM, Basket MM, Stokley SK, Dong F, Babbel CI, Seewald LA, Dickinson LM. Prevalence of parental concerns

about childhood vaccines: the experience of primary care physicians. Am J Prev Med. 2011;40(5):548–55.

50. Phadke VK, Bednarczyk RA, Salmon DA, Omer SB. Association between vaccine refusal and vaccine-preventable diseases in the United States: a review of measles and pertussis. JAMA. 2016;315(11):1149–58.

51. Attwell K, Ward P, Meyer SB, Rokkas PJ, Leask J. "Do-it-yourself": vaccine rejection and complementary and alternative medicine (CAM). Soc Sci Med. 2017;196. https://doi.org/10.1016/j.socscimed.2017.11.022.

52. Olive JK, Hotez PJ, Damania A, Nolan MS. The state of the antivaccine movement in the United States: a focused examination of nonmedical exemptions in states and counties. PLoS Med. 2018;15(6):e1002578. https://doi.org/10.1371/journal.pmed.1002578.

53. Hall V, Banerjee E, Kenyon C, et al. Measles outbreak—Minnesota April–may 2017. MMWR Morb Mortal Wkly Rep. 2017;66:713–7. https://doi.org/10.15585/mmwr.mm6627a1.

54. Levine A. NY Times. New York Today: Measles in Brooklyn. Oct 22, 2018.

55. National Academies of Sciences, Engineering, and Medicine. In: Gadsden VL, Ford M, Breiner H, editors. Parenting matters: supporting parents of children ages 0–8. Washington, DC: The National Academies Press; 2016. https://doi.org/10.17226/21868.

56. Ames HM, Glenton C, Lewin S. Parents' and informal caregivers' views and experiences of communication about routine childhood vaccination: a synthesis of qualitative evidence. Cochrane Database Syst Rev. 2017;2(2):CD011787. d.

57. http://www.who.int/immunization/programmes_systems/vaccine_hesitancy/en/).

58. Leask J, Kinnersley P, Jackson C, Cheater F, Bedford H, Rowles G. Communicating with parents about vaccination: a framework for health professionals. BMC Pediatr. 2012;12:154. https://doi.org/10.1186/1471-2431-12-154.

59. https://www.pm360online.com/motivational-interviewing-for-hpv-vaccination-well-accepted-by-doctors/.

Index

© Springer Nature Switzerland AG 2019   179
D. Huremović (ed.), *Psychiatry of Pandemics*,
https://doi.org/10.1007/978-3-030-15346-5